Systems of Care, The New Community Psychia... ... San Francisco:
Jossey-Bass.

Ireys, H.T., Devet, K.A., & Sakwa, D. (2002). Family support and education. In Burns,
J. & Hoagwood, K. (Eds.), *Community Treatment for Youth* (pp. 154-176). NY:
Oxford University Press.

Jackson, L.L., & Arbesman, M. (2005). *Occupational therapy practice guidelines for
children with behavioral and psychosocial needs*. Bethesda: American Occupational Therapy Association.

Kardos, M.R., & White, B.P. (2006). Evaluation options for secondary transition planning. *American Journal of Occupational Therapy, 60*(3), 333-339.

Knitzer, J. (2005). Advocacy for children's mental health: *A personal journey. Journal
of Clinical Child and Adolescent Psychology, 34*(4), 612-618.

Law, M., King, S., Stewart, D., & King, G. (2001). The perceived effects of parent-led
support groups for parents of children with disabilities. *Physical and Occupational
Therapy in Pediatrics, 21,* 29-48.

Lee, S.N., Gargiullo, A., Brayman, S., Kinsey, J.C., Jones, H.C., & Shotwell, M.
(2003). Adolescent performance on the Allen cognitive Levels Screen. *American
Journal of Occupational Therapy, 57*(3), 342-356.

Lourie, I.S., & Hernandez, M. (2003). A historical perspective on national child mental
health policy. *Journal of Emotional and Behavioral Disorders, 11*(1), 5-9.

McGinty, K.L., Diamond, J.M., Brown, M.B., & McCammon, S.L. (2003). Training
child and adolescent psychiatrists and child mental health professionals for systems
of care. In Pumariega, A.J. & Winters, N.C. (Eds.), *The Handbook of Child and Adolescent Systems of Care, The New Community Psychiatry* (pp. 487-507). San
Francisco: Jossey-Bass.

Meyers, J.C. (1985). Federal efforts to improve mental health services for children:
Breaking a cycle of failure. *Journal of Clinical Child Psychiatry, 14*(3), 182-187.

National Dissemination Center for Children with Disabilities. (2004). Emotional disturbance fact sheet 5. Retrieved March 19, 2007 from http://www.nichcy.org/
pubs/factshe/fs5txt.htm

Nolan, C., & Swarbrick, P. (2002). Supportive housing occupational therapy home
management program. *Mental Health Special Interest Section Quarterly, 25*(2),
1-3.

Olson, L.J. (2001). Child psychiatry in the USA. In Lougher, L. (Ed.), *Occupational
Therapy for Child and Adolescent Mental Health* (pp. 173-191). London: Churchill
Livingstone.

Passmore, A. (2003). The occupation of leisure: Three typologies and their influence
on mental health in adolescents. *Occupational Therapy Journal of Research, 23,*
76-84.

Rebeiro, K.L. (2001). Enabling occupation: The importance of an affirming environment. *Canadian Journal of Occupational Therapy, 68,* 80-89.

Stroul, B. (2003). Systems of care. In Pumariega, A.J. & Winters, N.C. (Eds.), *The
Handbook of Child and Adolescent Systems of Care, The New Community Psychiatry*
(pp. 17-34). San Francisco: Jossey-Bass.

Substance Abuse and Mental Health Service Administration. (May 2006). *SAMHSA News
Release: Community-Based Care Leads to Meaningful Improvement for Children and*

Youth with Serious Mental Health Needs. Downloaded February 14, 2007 from: http://systemsofcare.samhsa.gov/news/nrindex.aspx

Werner Degrace, B. (2003). The issue is–Occupation-based and family-centered care: A challenge for current practice. *American Journal of Occupational Therapy, 54,* 347-350.

Wooster, D.A. (2001). Early intervention programs. In Scaffa, M. (Ed.), *Occupational Therapy in Community-Based Practice Settings* (pp. 280-283). Philadelphia: F.A. Davis Company.

Zimmerman, S.S. (1999). Occupational therapy service delivery to an apartment program. *Home and Community Health Special Interest Section Quarterly, 6*(1), 1-4.

About the Contributors

Michael L. Burford, MSSW, is a PhD Student at the College of Social Work, The University of Tennessee.

Lyle Cooper, PhD, LCSW, earned his degree in Social Work from Spalding University. He is Assistant Professor at the College of Social Work, The University of Tennessee. He is also a Licensed Clinical Social Worker and a Certified Alcohol and Drug Counselor.

Gary D. Ellis, PhD, earned his degree in higher education administration from the University of North Texas. He is currently Professor in the Department of Parks, Recreation and Tourism at the University of Utah.

Rebecca I. Estes, PhD, OTR/L, ATP, earned her degree in Occupational Therapy from Texas Women's University. She is Associate Professor and Chair, Department of Occupational Therapy, University of South Alabama.

Claudette Fette, OTR, CRC, is Founder of the Denton County Federation of Families in Denton County, TX.

Tammy Holmes, MA, earned her degree in Educational Psychology and Counseling Education from Tennessee Technological University. She is the Drug Court Coordinator for the Upper Cumberland Juvenile Drug Court, employed through the Upper Cumberland Community Service Agency.

Carole Lovell, PsyD, MSSW, LCSW, earned her PsyD from Southern California University for Professional Studies and her MSSW from the University of Tennessee. Licensed as a Clinical Social Worker in Tennessee, she is also the Program Director for the Personal Growth and Learning Center in Cookeville, TN.

Samuel A. MacMaster, PhD, MSSA, earned his degrees from Case Western Reserve University. He is Associate Professor at the College of Social Work, The University of Tennessee.

William R. Nugent, PhD, MSSW, earned his degrees from Florida State University. He is Professor and Director of the Doctoral Program at the College of Social Work, The University of Tennessee, Knoxville.

Marjorie E. Scaffa, PhD, OTR/L, FAOTA, earned her degree in Health Education from the University of Maryland. She is Professor at the Department of Occupational Therapy, the University of South Alabama.

Karen M. Sowers, PhD, is Dean and Professor at the University of Tennessee College of Social Work in Knoxville.

Lori K. Holleran Stiker, PhD, MSW, ACSW, earned her PhD from Arizona State University and a MSW from the University of Pennsylvania. She is Associate Professor in the School of Social Work at the University of Texas, Austin.

Gregory Washington, PhD, MSW, LCSW, earned his degrees from Clark Atlanta University. He is Associate Professor at the University of Tennessee at Martin.

Jerry Watson, PhD, earned his degree in Urban Higher Education from Jackson State University. He is Assistant Vice President and Director of Housing and e-City Development for Jackson State University.

Roderick J. Watts, PhD, earned his degree from the University of Maryland, College Park. He is Associate Professor of Psychology at Georgia State University. He is also a member of the Community and Clinical Psychology Program

John Wodarski, PhD, MSSW, earned his PhD from Washington University and a MSSW from The University of Tennessee. He is Professor at the College of Social Work at The University of Tennessee.

Julie Worley, FNP, PMHNP, holds a Masters Degree in family practice from University of Illinois Chicago and a psychiatric nurse practitioner degree from University of South Alabama. She is a Family and Psychiatric Mental Health Nurse Practitioner with fifteen years experience as an advanced practice nurse and ten prior years experience as an RN. She is affiliated with the Personal Growth and Learning Center in Cookesville, TN.

Erik Yost, MS, earned his degree from the University of Utah. He also holds a BFA in advertising design from Syracuse University.

Index

Numbers followed by t indicate tables.

Best Practices in Residential Treatment

Best Practices in Residential Treatment is a detailed examination of the latest information on empirically tested, evidence-based interventions and procedures across the many dimensions of residential treatment practice. Respected authorities from a broad range of professions provide a truly interdisciplinary look into the various diverse aspects of the treatment of children and youths in a residential setting. The book brings the most current information available on best practices, cultural competence, substance abuse, facility management, medication management, and planning for community reentry.

This book provides the latest in research and practical techniques for the unique treatment program. This helpful resource extensively discusses effective counseling interventions, medication management approaches, facility management issues, and aftercare approaches to ensure successful outcomes for children and adolescents leaving a facility. The book's comprehensive nature offers practitioners the most current information on best practices in the residential treatment arena and can serve as a useful resource for future decision-making. This volume is extensively referenced and includes tables to clearly present data.

This book is a valuable resource for social workers, psychologists, psychiatrists, counselors, residential program administrators, state departments of children's services, educators, and students at all levels.

This book was published as a special issue of *Residential Treatment For Children & Youth.*

Rodney A. Ellis is Associate Professor of Social Work at the University of Tennessee and in clinical practice at Personal Growth and Learning Center, Cookeville, Tennessee. His areas of expertise include juvenile justice, child welfare, and cultural competence. He has practical treatment experience in numerous settings. He has also authored numerous studies, professional articles, and books.

Best Practices in Residential Treatment

Edited by Rodney A. Ellis

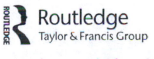

Routledge
Taylor & Francis Group

London and New York

First published 2009 by Routledge
2 Park Square, Milton Park, Abingdon, Oxon, OX14 4RN

Simultaneously published in the USA and Canada
by Routledge
270 Madison Avenue, New York, NY 10016

Routledge is an imprint of the Taylor & Francis Group, an Informa business

© 2009 Edited by Rodney A. Ellis

Typeset in Times by Value Chain, India
Printed and bound in the United States of America on acid-free paper by IBT Global

British Library Cataloguing in Publication Data
A catalogue record for this book is available from the British Library

ISBN10: 0-7890-3788-2 (h/b)
ISBN10: 0-7890-3789-0 (p/b)
ISBN13: 978-0-7890-3788-6 (h/b)
ISBN13: 978-0-7890-3789-3 (p/b)

CONTENTS

Foreword

Residential programs for children and adolescents are in flux. Concerns about effectiveness, cost and child safety have stimulated much public debate. Health care and human service professionals are facing greater demands for efficacious service than ever before. Previously accepted practice priorities are being questioned and accreditation bodies and third party reimbursers are challenging residential treatment systems to provide the highest standards of care, placing patient safety and accountability of patient progress at the core of practice. The pressure of responding to a managed care environment which challenges service providers to contain costs and document the application of best practices and evidence-based practice applications requires residential administrators and practitioners to continuously identify and apply cutting edge protocols and evidence-based practices within their practice environments. This is no easy task. The knowledge base on practice effectiveness is changing rapidly. Unfortunately, even with technological innovations and advancements, the ability to keep abreast of this growing body of knowledge can be overwhelming and daunting. Equally challenging is the ability of service providers to become trained and retrained in these new intervention technologies. The service provider must reframe their professional identity as one of "life long learner"–capable of adapting to change and the ability to incorporate new practice paradigms. Equally important is the service provider's commitment to engage in ongoing, systematic evaluation of practice effectiveness and use of evaluative findings to inform and improve practice.

Social institutions serving children and adolescents can positively or negatively impact outcomes on child and adolescent well being. The continual debates regarding institutional care and treatment for children and adolescents involve issues of cost, effectiveness, and presumed secondary social and psychological costs of the service. Despite the ongoing debates and challenges for residential treatment, there are a significant and disturbing number of children in need of residential services. Children and adolescents entering residential care settings exhibit a range of problems, including substance abuse, serious emotional disturbances, delinquent behaviors and learning and developmental disabilities. Increasingly children and adolescents are exhibiting multiple and co-occurring disorders and problems placing even greater challenges on treatment facilities.

This book is devoted to best practices in residential treatment for children and adolescents. It highlights the recent advances and trends in child and adolescent residential treatment. Its emphasis on interdisciplinary fields of practice is critically important as recent research findings underscore the need for a holistic approach to practice with interdisciplinary teams working together in an environment of mutual respect to coordinate services to meet all needs of the resident. This can only occur when there is an understanding of the roles and skills brought by each professional. An effective therapeutic milieu depends upon an integrated interdisciplinary approach.

The information highlighted in this book represents important contributions for service provision in residential treatment facilities for children and adolescents. In addition to the interdisciplinary approach to treatment, the book provides a critically important section on culture. To improve effectiveness we must be keenly aware of how developmental factors interact with environmental and cultural factors and how that interaction may alter or exacerbate problems. There is, however, a paucity of research on the development of minority and poor adolescents. The majority of intervention research has neglected issues of race, culture, sexual orientation and socio-economic status. Addressing the impact of various sociocultural factors on an individual's behavior, values, and beliefs may lead to more promising and effective approaches. And, as pointed out in this section, we must begin to view culture more broadly and in concert with the adolescent population itself.

The last section of this book focuses on community re-entry from residential treatment. This is perhaps the most challenging aspect of effective and sustainable treatment. Unless issues in the environment, including the family, peers and community are addressed, children and adolescents (who were successful in residential treatment) are highly likely to relapse. A seamless system of care from residential to community is critical to sustain initial treatment outcomes. This requires not only interdisciplinary approaches to community based care but a high level of interagency cooperation and coordination.

This is an exciting time for those of us who work in the field of services to children and adolescents and their families. New and emerging knowledge to inform our practice can provide us with the foundation for treatments for children and adolescents which are effective and sustainable. Research evidence challenges us to open ourselves to new technologies, to new interdisciplinary collaborations and to the development of specific interventions which are culturally sensitive and responsive. *Best Practices in Residential Treatment* is bursting with valuable information which will benefit practitioners, administrators, and policy makers. It makes a significant contribution to our understanding of issues in residential treatment for children and youth and provides us with a roadmap for the future. There can be no more important work than that which strengthens the productivity and health of our youth.

Karen M. Sowers, PhD
Dean and Professor
The University of Tennessee
College of Social Work

Introduction

Rodney A. Ellis, PhD, CMSW

This volume was conceived as an opportunity to update practitioners, researchers, administrators, and policy makers on recent advances and trends in child and adolescent residential treatment. Although it remains to be seen what others will learn from it, its editor has learned a great deal. The intent was to solicit papers from experts in specific dimensions of the field, areas like best practices, substance abuse, facility management, medication management, cultural competence, and planning for community re-entry. As I heard from the experts, I learned that many changes have occurred in many areas, yet very little is different in many others.

Another goal for the collection was that it be cross-disciplinary. Some may be surprised to find such diverse fields as psychiatric nursing, recreation, and occupational therapy, and will doubtless be pleased by the contributors they bring. It is easy to become insular, reading only the writings of those easily discerned as our colleagues when, in fact, our circle of colleagues may be broader than we think.

Each article in this volume addresses at least one dimension of residential treatment. The first three articles deal with best practices and promising practices in residential treatment. Eric Yost, PhD and Gary

Ellis, PhD, faculty from the field of recreation, both very interested in its application for prevention and treatment, report the results of an outcome study in which self determination theory-based recreational activities were used in a treatment program. That is followed by an article by Carole Lovelle, a practitioner who unites social work and psychology with her MSSW and PsyD. Carole makes a case for using Dialectical Behavior therapy concurrently with Eye Movement Desensitization and Reprocessing to treat adolescents with trauma-related issues. She has dones so in her own practice with great success and points to evidence both empirical and logical of its potential effectiveness. The third article, by two social workers and an educational psychologist (Sam MacMaster, PhD, the current writer, and Tammy Holmes, MA) reports the results of an outcome study of a juvenile drug court and discusses possibilities of combining that intervention with residential treatment. These constitute the contributions to the dimension of treatment.

Culture and cultural sensitivity are increasingly important to residential treatment. Two articles address this topic. One, written by Lori Holleran Steiker, PhD, an associate professor of social work, is a thought-provoking, comprehensive look at the many levels and forms of culture within a facility. The second, penned by Gregory Washington, PhD, Roderick Watts, PhD, and Jerry Watson, PhD (also social workers) reports the results of a single experience with Man Seekers Camp, a residential camping intervention for African American youth.

Advances in treating mental illnesses with psychotropic medication are discussed in the sixth article, written by Julie Worley, FNP, PMHNP. She is in practice as a clinical nurse practitioner working with children and adolescents in both inpatient and outpatient settings. Ms. Worley's article reviews current treatment alternatives for many of the major psychiatric conditions experienced by children and adolescents and describes some of the possible side effects of each.

Two articles consider facility management. The first describes the results of a study by Mike Burford, MSSW (a PhD student), William Nugent, PhD, and John Wodarski, PhD. The study sought to determine whether off-campus passes with an adult mentor or family member helped to decrease the probability of elopement from treatment. The second, by Sam MacMaster, PhD, Lyle Cooper, PhD, and the present writer, discusses issues of facility functioning and survival in a post-managed care era.

The final article focuses on aftercare. Rebecca Estes, PhD, ORT/L, ATP, Claudette Fette, OTR, CRC, the Founder of Denton County Federation of Families, Texas, and Marjorie E. Scaffa, PhD, OTR/L, FAOTA, all occupational therapists, offer a contribution discussing techniques that can facilitate successful reentry for children and adolescents leaving residential treatment.

Hopefully, readers will find the diversity of content interesting, informative, and helpful. It certainly has been to me.

Effect of Self Determination Theory-Based Recreation Activity-Staging on Vitality and Affinity Toward Nature Among Youth in a Residential Treatment Program

Erik Yost, MS
Gary D. Ellis, PhD

INTRODUCTION

A major challenge in working with youth who have behavioral, emotional, and learning disabilities is staging environments and activities that fully engage participants in tasks at hand, rather than leaving them detached and disaffected (Skinner, 2002, p. 299; Patrick, Skinner, & Connell, 1993; Wellborn, 1991). Little is known, however, of specific techniques that reliably elicit engagement. The practice of staging experiences that have transformational potential for youth (Pine & Gilmore, 1999; Ralston, Ellis, Compton, & Lee, 2006) remains much more art than science (Long, Ellis, Trunnell, Tatsugawa, & Freeman, 2001; Rossman & Schlatter, 2000). Self-determination theory (Deci & Ryan, 1985; 2002; Reeve, Bolt, & Cai, 1999) suggests a number of principles that might be used by adult activity leaders to elicit target emotional and motivational states among youth. This study thus examined the effect of a recreation activity staged according to self-determination theory principles on situational vitality and affinity for nature of male high school students in a residential treatment facility. The staging strategies were constructed to engage and satisfy psychological needs for autonomy, competence, and relatedness (Deci & Ryan, 2002; Deci, Eghrari, Patrick, & Leone, 1994; Deci, Ryan, & Williams, 1996; Ryan & Deci, 2000) during a snow-shoe tour. The rationale for the investigation follows.

RATIONALE

Engagement refers to "active, goal-directed, flexible, constructive, persistent, focused interactions with the social and physical environment" (Skinner, 2002, p. 299). In contrast, "disaffected actions" are present when individuals are emotionally and behaviorally alienated from participation" in activities (Skinner, 2002; Patrick, Skinner, & Connell, 1993; Wellborn, 1991). Engagement provides an important foundation for learning specific skills, habits, behaviors, and values. It is a necessary condition for the implementation fidelity (Domitrovich & Greenberg, 2000; Duesnbury, Brannigan, Falco, & Hansen, 2003) and thus outcome efficacy of interventions. The ability to apply techniques for eliciting and sustaining engagement is thus an important skill for youth service professionals in a variety of settings.

Self-determination theory (SDT; Deci & Ryan, 1985; Deci & Ryan, 2002; Ryan & Deci, 2000) offers a number of principles that have notable potential for eliciting engagement. Engagement is a function of activation of psychological needs and satisfaction of those needs (Reeve, 2004). SDT proposes three organismic psychological needs that are inherent in all people: the need for autonomy, the need for competence, and the need for relatedness. These psychological needs are assumed to parallel such tissue-deficit needs as hunger, thirst, temperature regulation, and sexual activity in that, like these physiological needs, inattention to psychological needs results in significant and serious dysfunction. Psychological needs are particularly relevant to the challenge of engaging youth in activity, because circumstances that serve to satisfy such needs are experienced as engaging: "When an activity involves our psychological needs, we feel interest [and] when an activity satisfies our psychological needs, we feel enjoyment" (Reeve, 2004, p. 102). Within SDT, the subjective experience of having psychological needs met is called in-situ (state) "vitality" (Nix, Ryan, Manly, & Deci, 1999; Ryan & Frederick, 1997; Kasser & Ryan, 1993).

In addition to in-situ vitality, research has shown that affinity toward nature can create a number of positive outcomes for youth. Affinity toward nature refers to the cognitive value judgment that drives one's emotional response toward nature (Nussbaum, 2001; Solomon, 1988). Among the many benefits that have been found to result from contacts with natural environments are help in counteracting attention difficulties (Kaplan, Kaplan, & Ryan, 1998; Taylor, Kuo, & Sullivan, 2001); alleviating depression, stress, and anxiety (Kahn, 1999; Wells & Evans, 2003); assistance in fostering concentration (Taylor, Kuo, & Sullivan, 2002), promoting growth and development (Moore, 1997), and stimulating creativity (Cobb, 1977; Chawla, 1986).

It is reasonable to propose that in-situ vitality and affinity toward nature may result from situations that engage and satisfy psychological needs for autonomy, competence, and relatedness among youth (Deci & Ryan, 1985; 2002; Reeve, 2004, p. 102). By eliciting in-situ vitality through engagement of psychological needs in natural settings, positive associations between the quality of immediate experiences and the natural environment could be expected to occur. These associations may, in turn, facilitate in-situ affinity for nature. Existing research supports the position that activity staging techniques may successfully be used to engage and satisfy psychological needs. Long, Ellis, Trunnell, Tatsugawa, and Freeman (2001), for example, found that recreation activity staging techniques that are designed to elicit situational feelings of competence elicit enjoyment, self-efficacy, and positivity of affect. Results that are consistent with these occurred in a study that involved experiences staged to engage both competence and relatedness needs (Roark & Ellis, 2007). Other studies have identified effective strategies that can be used to stage experiences that elicit target emotional and motivational states, conceptual learning, and pro-environmental behaviors (Garbarino, 1975; Patrick, Skinner, & Connell, 1993; Koestner, Ryan, Bernieri, & Holt, 1984; Grolnick & Ryan, 1987; Legault & Pelletier, 2000). These studies provide compelling evidence that specific techniques may be used to stage encounters that engage the psychological needs of autonomy, competence, and relatedness that are advanced by self-determination theory (Deci & Ryan, 1985; 2002).

No studies have been completed, however, that directly address the effect of SDT-based activity staging strategies on in-situ vitality and affinity toward nature. The activity staging strategies that have been demonstrated to be effective in other recreation and education settings and contexts may be insufficient to create change in participants' evaluations in the natural environment. The novelties and complexities of the natural environment may be sufficient, in and of themselves, to affect affinity toward nature. Wilson (1984), in fact, proposes that humans possess an innate tendency toward nature. Nature, according to Wilson, is inherent in human beings and nature encounters are naturally pleasing. Individual and cultural differences also play a role in how emotions are construed (Ortony, Clore, & Collins, 1988). These differences may work against any efforts put forth by instructors in executing staging strategies.

Further, it is notable that most students who attend residential treatment programs do so against their will, resulting in a generalized state of either external motivation or amotivation (Deci & Ryan, 2002) among the students. Psychological needs are best met, however, through engagements that are characterized by intrinsic motivation (Deci & Ryan, 1985, 2002). Activity staging strategies aimed at meeting autonomy, competence, and relatedness needs may thus be insufficient to create identified, integrated, or intrinsic value toward nature in students in residential treatment programs.

Further, students in residential treatment programs struggle with a variety of issues, such as unresolved trauma, depression, anxiety, oppositional behaviors, impulsivity and attention difficulties, social, self-esteem, and relationship difficulties, substance abuse, identity and developmental difficulties, and academic and learning disabilities. Facilitating satisfaction of the basic psychological needs of autonomy, competence, and relatedness might prove to be a daunting task, given the host of difficulties these students face. In addition, it is notable that students in residential treatment live, attend school, and undergo therapy together. Participants thus have a wealth of opportunities to connect with social structures that meet relatedness needs. Activity staging strategies in a recreation environment may perceived by students as trivial fractions of environments that are already highly stimulating. If so, such strategies could not be expected to significantly enhance vitality through activation and meeting of psychological needs.

Fear may also intercede. Fear is a common emotion associated with natural areas (Bixler & Floyd, 1997; Bixler, Carlisle, Hammitt, & Floyd, 1994; Wohlwill, 1974). It creates significant barriers to individuals' contacts with nature. The cognitive aspect of fear has been described as the associations of feared objects with places and situations in which they may be encountered (Bixler, Floyd, & Hammitt, 1995). These negative associations of nature affect the value judgments that individuals make toward nature.

Thus, SDT theory points to strategies for staging recreation encounters that may elicit vitality and affinity for nature. Other evidence suggests that any effect from such mechanisms may be overshadowed by more powerful personal and contextual factors. The purpose of this study, therefore, was to examine the effect of a SDT-based recreation activity staging strategy on vitality and affinity toward nature among teen-age male students enrolled in a residential treatment program.

METHOD

Participants

Two hundred fifty-two observations were gathered from 21, 14-17 year old students enrolled in an all-male residential treatment program in Utah. Students of that program face a variety of behavioral, emotional, learning, and dependency issues. The admissions criteria for the program describe underachieving boys struggling with unresolved trauma, depression, anxiety, oppositional behaviors, impulsivity and attention problems, social problems, diminished self-esteem, substance abuse, difficulties at home, relationship problems, identity and developmental issues, academic deficits, and other comparable difficulties. Contraindications for admission include youth who present with imminently life threatening symptoms, pose a danger to self or others, present a history of chronic substance abuse without a recent intervening period of sobriety, present as physically aggressive, or require extreme physical or medical care.

The average length of stay for students enrolled in the treatment program is seven to nine months. In practice, length of stay is highly flexible and is based on the needs and progress of the individual student. The program maxim is that every student receives an individualized balance of intense therapy, demanding schooling in accredited high school curricula, and structured therapeutic recreation.

The treatment facility was designed to provide a home-like environment. The program is directed by its owners, and direct leadership to students is provided by highly credentialed, licensed clinicians. Four full-time licensed therapists work directly with students to provide and execute individualized and family therapy plans. Each participant is a member of a peer group of students with whom the individual participates in daily functions such as meals, chores, recreation, and clinical/ therapeutic groups. An integrated weekend therapeutic recreation component includes a snowshoeing component. Other outdoor recreation activities that occur on separate tours as a part of the recreation program include rock climbing, hiking, camping, backpacking, rafting, and skiing/snowboarding.

Measurement

Students were asked to complete measures of in-situ vitality and affinity toward nature on six occasions during each of two snowshoe tours (SDT-staged and traditional). Facilitating staff were instructed to administer the remaining questionnaires over the time that participants were actually in the field, according to a timeline provided. One questionnaire, for example, was completed at the trailhead, another was completed before the environmental education lesson began, and the final questionnaire was completed following the activity, back at the trailhead.

The questionnaire for measuring these two concepts included a total of 14 bipolar adjectives. Eight of these were chosen to measure affinity for nature. These items were selected from the "evaluation" dimension of Osgood, Suci, and Tannenbaum's (1957) classic research on measurement of meaning. Six bipolar adjective pairs were used to measure in-situ vitality. A visual analog response format was used for both measures. Each pair of adjectives was separated by a 100 mm line, and students were asked to mark the point on that line that best represented their experience at the moment that immediately preceded the time that they were asked to complete the questionnaire. Response units were millimeters from the negative end of the scale (i.e., low in-situ vitality and low in-situ affinity for nature). The visual analog format was pre-tested with this group prior to collecting data, and students indicated full understanding of the expectations of the method.

In-Situ Vitality

The eight items used to measure in-situ vitality were drawn from the subjective vitality scale. The specific bipolar pairs of in-situ vitality indictors were: alive vs. bored to death, important vs. unimportant, tired vs. energetic, lifeless vs. spirited, alert vs. sluggish, and asleep vs. awake. Three of these indicator pairs were reverse ordered to reduce the possibility of a response set bias. The meaning of each word and the response format was discussed with students prior to the two tours. The alpha reliability of this six-item measure was .91.

Affinity Toward Nature

Affinity toward nature was measured through eight bipolar adjectives: good vs. bad, beautiful vs. ugly, uncomfortable vs. comfortable, meaningful vs. meaningless, unimportant vs. important, repelling vs. attracting, positive vs. negative, and appealing vs. offensive. Students were asked to place a mark on the 100 mm line that "represents your judgment of nature and of your feelings at this moment." Like the items on the in-situ vitality scale, the meaning of the words used on the affinity toward nature scale was discussed with students prior to the first tour. The alpha reliability of this eight-item measure was .95.

Procedure

All snowshoe tours occurred in the Wasatch Mountains of north central Utah. The Wasatch Mountains offer many opportunities for snowshoeing and other winter sports. Trails were selected carefully, with consideration of initial elevation (8,000 to 10,000 feet), elevation gains, terrain, length, and other features, in order to optimize the level of challenge for the students. All tours were day trips lasting approximately 4-6 hours. Snowshoeing is a standard part of the recreation program for the students, but none of the students on these tours had participated in snow-shoeing previously.

Each three cohorts of students participated in snowshoe tours on two consecutive weekends. One of these tours was staged using principles designed to engage and satisfy psychological needs for autonomy, competence, and relatedness. The other tour was a traditional recreational "competent tutor" snowshoe tour, with emphasis on successful execution of skills required for the activity, but no unique attempt by adult leaders to engage psychological needs (Bishop & Jenrenaud, 1995). The design was counter-balanced to allow for the testing of the carry-over effect. One group of students received the staged tour during the first week-end of the program, and then participated in the traditional tour on the following week-end. The other two groups followed the opposite pattern.

Although counterbalancing is typically used to control extraneous variance related to treatment order, in this investigation treatment order was central to the study purpose. We reasoned that students who received the staged tour first could quite possibly learn techniques that they could apply to meet psychological needs on subsequent tours, apart from techniques used by leaders. In addition, in-situ affinity for nature that results from positive association with a tour might generalize to a more generalized evaluation of nature on subsequent tours. As such, students who received the staged experience first might be expected to show greater in-situ affinity for nature during their second tour, as a function of the staging mechanisms they experienced during the tour of the previous week. For these reasons, a treatment-by-treatment order interaction was hypothesized with respect to both in-situ vitality and in-situ affinity for nature.

SDT-Staged Tours

The SDT-staged tours involved execution of techniques derived from self-determination theory (Deci & Ryan, 1985, 2002). As such, students' needs for autonomy, competence, and relatedness needs were targeted through specific leadership strategies employed during the course of the tour. Table 1 provides a detailed description of the strategies used to engage and satisfy students' psychological needs during the SDT-Staged tours.

Examples of techniques that were used to engage the competence need are use of structure, optimal challenge, failure tolerance, competence feedback messages, informational feedback messages, and praise. Relatedness was addressed by fostering communal relationships. All of the activities on these tours were conducted in a social environment of autonomy-support. Autonomy-support was facilitated by intense and non-judgmental listening, perspective-taking, providing a rationale for decisions, encouraging effort, and providing meaningful choice among

TABLE 1. Techniques Used to Engage and Satisfy Students' Psychological Needs During SDT Tour

Tour Phase	Psychological Need	Technique
Pre-tour preparation	Autonomy	Interests, preferences, and competencies were identified through discussions with students. Member checking was used to confirm correct identification of these identity-relevant characteristics.
Pre-tour preparation	Autonomy	The value, worth, meaning, utility, or importance for engagement in activities was communicated to the student through a conversation involving staff and students.
Pre & During tour	Autonomy	When instances of conflict or expression of negative affect occurred, staff listened carefully and accepted negative reactions as valid. Staff used established SDT mechanisms: perspective taking, reasoning, and choice.
During tour	Autonomy	Staff used informational language rather than controlling language to provide feedback and to address motivational and/or behavioral difficulties.
During tour	Competence	Staff staged the encounter with opportunity for optimal challenge, given each individual's ability.
During tour	Competence	Staff staged social contexts that were tolerant of failure and difficulty. This was accomplished by supporting engagement; encouraging learning from failure; valuing failure as a learning and growth opportunity; and supporting competence and mastery of challenge.
Pre & During tour	Competence	Structure provides support and guidance. Staff directly modeled, explained, coached, and taught each student. Staff also allowed for other, more competent students to teach those students who were struggling. Staff explained problem-solving strategies, communicated expectations, helped regulate negative emotions, and shared insight on repairing and preventing negative outcomes.
During tour	Competence	Competence messages in the form of informational feedback were delivered by staff. Such messages are more effective than ambiguous and/or controlling messages at increasing perceived competence.
During & Post-tour	Competence	Praise was included as a positive feedback technique. This approach has been demonstrated to be particularly powerful when used with males.
Pre, During, & Post-tour	Relatedness	Staff facilitated relationships and interactions in ways that promoted caring, liking, acceptance, and valuing between students.
Pre, During, & Post-tour	Relatedness	Staff fostered communal relationships by facilitating checking in about the needs of others, avoiding competition, reciprocity, material gain, and individualism, and providing help for distressed individuals.

options relevant to students' interests, preferences, and competencies (Reeve, 2005).

To establish the personal relevance necessary for intrinsically motivating experiences, students were asked to choose a meaningful activity to do while on the SDT-based snowshoe tour. One student, for example, had special interest in photography, so his tour involved collecting photographic images of nature that would be suitable for a computer "screen-saver." An environmental education lesson also was part of the tour; instructors taught students about different animal tracks and gaits. During the SDT tour, students were given a meaningful choice opportunity; they were asked to chose an animal to which they could most relate, create a set of tracks in the snow representing a path that animal had followed, and craft a story involving the tracks.

Competence messages were designed in accordance with research within SDT concerning positive, informational feedback. Feedback that is informational as opposed to evaluation-based is more effective in increasing perceived competence (Deci & Ryan, 1985). Trip leaders were thus trained to frame feedback concerning competence in an informational rather than evaluative way during the SDT-based tour. For example: "when the straps on a snowshoe are tight the shoe won't fall off as easily" (informational) versus "you haven't strapped the snowshoe on tight enough so it won't stay on well" (evaluational).

An exception to use of competence messages as evaluational is made for opportunities for praise. Praise has been shown to be more effective when working with boys than with girls (Deci & Ryan, 1985). Even though it is a form of evaluative feedback, it is positive and thus supports the perceived competence of the male student (e.g., "You are a very strong snowshoer!" "You are good at getting the snowshoe on!" "You get up quickly after you fall!"). When praising, the attention must necessarily be directed at the person and be positive.

To create feelings of relatedness, students were encouraged to work in small groups during the choice activity and during animal track activity, except when working in groups was inconsistent with the autonomous choice of a particular student. Small groups with no more than three or four students were formed for this purpose. Instructors also facilitated a discussion beforehand that focused on the group as a whole. During that discussion, they asked "What do you hope to contribute to the group today?" and "How does it feel to be part of the snowshoeing group?"

Instructors were trained through a formal introduction to self-determination theory and its tenants, as well as by actually going into the field to do a simulated tour. During the simulated tour, trip leaders practiced facilitating autonomy, competence, and relatedness while other leaders role-played students.

Traditional Tour

The traditional tours were conducted in a manner that was as similar as possible to how snowshoe tours had been conducted on tours of previous years, involving other groups of students. These tours involved focus on snowshoeing skills, and they included typical interactions among students and tour leaders. Although students were in groups during these tours, no efforts were made by leaders to accentuate relatedness among those participants. No meaningful choice activity was part of the traditional snowshoe experience, and scripted competence messages that were provided during the SDT-based tour were not given during the traditional tour. No effort was made, however, to withhold feedback messages that would typically be given or in any other way to diminish the quality of the experience of students. This approach approximates the "competent tutor" model for staging experiences that has been used in previous research (Bishop & Jenrenaud, 1985; Long et al., 2001). Because both the traditional and SDT-based models seek to create positive experiences for participants, key similarities and differences exist. Figure 1 provides a description of these similarities and differences, using a Venn diagram.

Data Analysis

Data were analyzed separately for the two outcome variables. Means and standard deviations were calculated for each of the treatment conditions defined by tour type (SDT-based vs. traditional) and treatment order (SDT-based tour first vs. traditional tour first). The significance of the effect of treatment, treatment order, and their interaction was tested using hierarchical linear modeling (Radenbush & Bryk, 2002). That approach

FIGURE 1. Similarities and differences between experimental and traditional or non-treatment conditions.

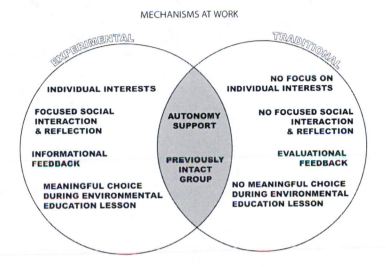

MECHANISMS AT WORK

EXPERIMENTAL

TRADITIONAL

INDIVIDUAL INTERESTS

FOCUSED SOCIAL
INTERACTION
& REFLECTION

INFORMATIONAL
FEEDBACK

MEANINGFUL CHOICE
DURING ENVIRONMENTAL
EDUCATION LESSON

AUTONOMY
SUPPORT

PREVIOUSLY
INTACT
GROUP

NO FOCUS ON
INDIVIDUAL INTERESTS

NO FOCUSED SOCIAL
INTERACTION
& REFLECTION

EVALUATIONAL
FEEDBACK

NO MEANINGFUL CHOICE
DURING ENVIRONMENTAL
EDUCATION LESSON

allows the dependency among observations to be modeled and it allows the variance to be partitioned between two or more levels (in this case, the in-situ experience level and the student level). In the model that was constructed, the 252 individual measurements of vitality and affinity toward nature were nested within the random effect of individual differences among the 21 student participants. For the Level 1 (in-situ experience) portion of the model, a centered dummy vector was constructed to represent the effect of tour type. Treatment order was a Level 2 variable (a characteristic of the student). That variable was also represented by a dummy variable in the model, and it was modeled on both the Level 1 intercept and the Level 1 slope of treatment to evaluate its main effect and (cross-level) interaction with treatment, respectively. The specific model tested for each of the two variables was the following:

Level 1

$$Y = \pi_0 + \pi_1(treatment) + e$$

Level 2

$$\pi_0 = \beta_{00} + \beta_{11}(order) + r_0$$

$$\pi_1 = \beta_{10} + \beta_{11}(order) + r_1$$

Association strength was measured through R^2_{PRE}, which is the reduction in variance from the models that included the dummy variables, as compared to a null (intercept only) model. The intraclass correlation was calculated from the null model to represent the proportion of variance that resulted from differences across students vs. differences in situations. Treatment condition means were plotted to facilitate interpretation of significant interaction effects.

RESULTS

Descriptive Statistics

TABLE 2. Treatment Condition Means and Standard Deviations

	Mean	SD	N
Vitality			
SDT-Staged Tour (Marginal)	61.11	23.06	126
SDT Tour First	73.72	17.38	42
Traditional Tour First	54.80	23.03	84
Traditional Tour (Marginal)	62.93	21.50	126
SDT Tour First	69.01	22.88	42
Traditional Tour First	59.89	20.24	84
Treatment Order Main Effects			
SDT Tour First	71.36	20.34	84
Traditional Tour First	57.35	21.77	168
Affinity Toward Nature			
SDT-Staged Tour (Marginal)	70.38	21.17	126
SDT Tour First	82.02	12.77	42
Traditional Tour First	64.56	22.17	84
Traditional Tour (Marginal)	71.17	19.03	126
SDT Tour First	77.53	15.37	42
Traditional Tour First	67.99	19.95	84
Treatment Order Main Effect			
SDT Tour First	79.77	14.22	84
Traditional Tour First	66.27	21.09	168

Treatment condition means and standard deviations are reported in Table 2. The largest mean for vitality was during the SDT-staged tour, when that tour was experienced first ($M = 73.72, SD = 17.38$). The lowest mean was also observed under the SDT-staged tour, when that tour occurred after the traditional tour ($M = 54.80, SD = 23.03$). The identical pattern occurred for affinity for nature. When the SDT-staged tour occurred first, the affinity toward nature mean was 82.02 ($SD = 12.77$), but when the SDT-staged tour was second in treatment order, the lowest treatment condition mean for affinity toward nature was observed, 64.56 ($SD = 22.17$). The smallest standard deviations for both vitality and affinity for nature ($SD = 17.38$ and 12.77, respectively) were observed when that the STD-staged tour was experienced first in the treatment order. Thus, the SDT-staged condition, when experienced by students first produced the highest means and the smallest standard deviations among the treatment conditions.

Also notable among the descriptive statistics is the similarity of marginal (main effect) means associated with STD-staged tours vs. traditional tours. For vitality, the means differed by only 1.82 units (62.93 minus 61.11), and for affinity toward nature, the means differed by only .79 units (71.17 minus 70.38). In both cases, the traditional tour mean was very slightly greater than the SDT-staged tour mean.

Overall, the patterns of means suggest an interaction effect. The SDT-staged tours produced the highest scores, but only when those tours were experienced first. When experienced second in the treatment order, the SDT-staged tours produced notably low scores on both vitality and affinity toward nature.

Hypothesis Tests

Tables 3 and 4 provide summaries of the hypothesis tests for each of the variables. The cross-level interaction effect was found to be significant for both vitality ($t_{248} = 2.18, p = .03$) and affinity toward nature ($t_{248} = 2.05, p = .041$). The tables also show a reduction in error variance of the alternative vs. the null model (R^2_{PRE}) of 8% for vitality and 9% for affinity toward nature. Intra-class correlations reveal that 43% of the variance in vitality was associated with individual differences among

TABLE 3. Hypothesis Test: Vitality

	Coef	SE	df	t	p
Vitality Fixed Effects					
For Intercept 1 (π_0)					
Intercept 2 (β_{00})	71.37	5.44	19	13.11	<.001
Treatment Order (β_{01})	−14.02	6.67	19	−2.10	.049
For Treatment (Staging Technique, π_1)					
Intercept 2 (β_{10})	−4.71	3.67	248	−1.29	.200
Treatment Order (β_{11})	9.81	4.49	248	2.18	.030
Random Effects	SD	Var Comp	df	χ^2	p
r_0	13.56	183.85	19	167.54	<.001
e	16.80	282.19			

$R^2_{PRE} = .08$
Null Model intraclass $r = .43$

TABLE 4. Hypothesis Test: Affinity for Nature

	Coef	SE	df	t	p
Affinity Toward Nature Fixed Effects					
For Intercept 1 (π_0)					
Intercept 2 (β_{00})	79.77	5.14	19	15.51	<.001
Treatment Order (β_{01})	−13.50	6.30	19	−2.14	.045
For Treatment (Staging Technique, π_1)					
Intercept 2 (β_{10})	−4.49	3.16	248	−1.42	.156
Treatment Order (β_{11})	7.91	3.87	248	2.05	.041
Random Effects	SD	Var Comp	df	χ^2	p
r_0	12.95	167.75	19	201.60	<.001
e	14.47	209.45			

$R^2_{PRE} = .09$
Null Model intraclass $r = .49$

students. For affinity toward nature, 49% of the variance was attributable to individual differences among students.

Plots (Figure 2) were constructed to facilitate interpretation of the significant interaction effects. Both interactions were found to be disordinal. For SDT-staged tours, the means of both dependent variables were high, but only for the group that experienced the SDT-staged tour first. The mean of the SDT-staged tour dropped dramatically for the two groups who experienced the SDT-staged tour on the week following the traditional tour. For the traditional tour conditions, the mean was highest when the SDT-staged tours were conducted first. When the traditional tours were conducted after the SDT-staged tours, the means dropped, but were higher than the means of the SDT-staged tours that were experienced second in treatment order.

DISCUSSION

This study sought to evaluate the effect of SDT-based activity staging on in-situ vitality and in-situ affinity toward nature among male youths in a residential treatment program. Results revealed a significant treatment-by-treatment order interaction for both of these outcomes. When the SDT-staged tour was experienced before the traditional tour, vitality and affinity toward nature were high. When the SDT-staged tour was experienced after having previously participated in a traditional tour, however, the means were dramatically lower. For the group that experienced the SDT-staged tour first, the traditional tour produced higher means than the SDT-staged tour.

FIGURE 2. Treatment (Tour Type) by treatment order (SDT-staged vs. traditional first) interactions

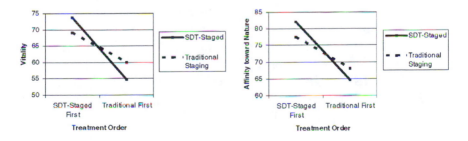

These results strongly suggest that, despite the presence of numerous social and contextual factors that may influence reactions of youth to interventions, significant learning tends to occur from one experience to the next. This observation is reflected in the fact that both the highest and lowest means occurred in the SDT-staged tours. The highest mean occurred among students who experienced the SDT-staged tour before experiencing the traditional tour. The lowest means occurred among students who experienced the SDT-staged tour as the second tour. A reasonable explanation for these results is that youth develop specific expectations for experiences on their initial tours. When those expectations are not met subsequently, the quality of the experience is significantly diminished. This explanation is fully consistent with the "discrepancy models" that have long been used to explain satisfaction with recreation experiences (e.g., Iso-Ahola, 1980; Mannell, 1989) and quality management models that explain customer satisfaction in terms of expectations with respect to quality (Pyzdek, 2003; Walden, 1993). Further, these results suggest the possibility that youth may learn important intrapersonal abilities through individual nature experiences of 4-6 hours in duration. These results are consistent with previous research that has evaluated SDT-related and SDT-based interventions in school (Deci, Kasser, & Ryan, 1997; Reeve, Bolt, & Cai, 1999; Grolnick & Ryan, 1987; Gabrino, 1975), camp (Hill & Sibthorp, 2006; Ramsing, 2005), and recreation (Roark & Ellis, 2007) settings. SDT-related techniques can be used to increase engagement, enhance learning, and facilitate development of affinity for activities that may contribute to development and socialization of youth.

A notable addition of these results to the literature on staging recreation experiences is the effect sizes. Effect sizes were larger in this study than those of similar studies in other settings. The effect sizes for vitality and affinity for nature were .08 and .09, respectively. Although these could not appropriately be categorized as "strong" effects, they are markedly larger than effect sizes reported previously. In studies of the effects of intentional programming toward target camp outcomes, for example, association strength measures (partial eta squared, eta squared) of less than .05 are typical (Ramsing, 2005; Hill & Sibthorp, 2006). These estimates are fully consistent with association strength measures that have been reported in studies of the effects of recreation activity staging strategies on in-situ measures of emotional and motivational states (Roark & Ellis, 2007; Long et al., 2001). Studies of the effects of the well-known task challenge by personal skill interaction on immediate conscious experiences (e.g., Csikszentmihlayi & Csikszentmihalyi, 1988) have also yielded association strength estimates of less than .05 (Ellis, Voelkl, & Morris, 1994).

The large intra-class correlation coefficients observed in this study clearly suggest the appropriateness of additional inquiry on staging experiences. For both variables, the percentage of variance attributable to individual differences among students exceeded .40. This, of course, indicates that the majority of the variance (approximately 60%) in in-situ experiences is a function of factors operative in the immediate, in-situ activity, task, and encounter of the individual student. Research is needed to identify they key agents of change that determine in-situ experiences of youth, along with ways to incorporate those agents into interventions directed at improving the lives of youth.

This study employed a complex "mix" of SDT-based agents to enhance experiences. Techniques included inclusion of special experiences that highlighted autonomy through meaningful choice, carefully staged performance feedback, structure, discussions, and SDT-based conflict resolution techniques (i.e., perspective-taking, rationale, and choice). Future research is needed to dissect this "black box" of techniques, so that leaders of youth activities can efficiently include a manageable number of strategies in their "toolkits" for working directly with youth. Future research might also address variation attributable to the random effect of individual differences between tour/activity/intervention leader (which was $R^2_{PRE} = .05$ in this study). At issue is the challenge of sustaining the fidelity of the intervention, given different interpersonal styles, experience levels, preparation, talent, and commitments of youth leaders and service providers. The weak association strength in this study suggests that the rigorous training regimen was effective. Unknown, however, are the specific components of the training that led to this result and what elements might be eliminated to achieve greater efficiency.

NOTE

This paper is based on masters thesis research of the first author.

REFERENCES

Bishop, D., & Jeanrenaud, C. (1995). Creative growth through play and its implications for recreation practice. In P. A. W. T. L. Goodale (Ed.), *Recreation and leisure: Issues in an era of change* (pp. 87-104). State College, PA: Venture Publishing.

Bixler, R. D., & Floyd, M. F. (1997). Nature is scary, disgusting, and uncomfortable. *Environment and Behavior, 29*(4), 443-467.

Bixler, R. D., Carlisle, C. L., Hammitt, W. E., & Floyd, M. F. (1994). Observed fears and discomforts among urban students on school field trips to wildland areas. *Journal of Environmental Education, 26*, 24-33.

Bixler, R. D., Floyd, M. F., & Hammitt, W. E. (1995). Feared stimuli are expected in specific situations: Using an expectancy approach and situationalism in self-report measures of fears. *Journal of Clinical Psychology, 51*, 544-547.

Chawla, L. (1986). The ecology of environmental memory. *Children's Environmental Quarterly, 3* (4), pp. 34-42.

Cobb, E. (1977). *The Ecology of Imagination in Childhood*. New York: Columbia University Press.

Csikszentmihalyi, M., & Csikszentmihalyi, I. S. (1988). *Optimal experience: Psychological studies of flow in consciousness*. New York, NY: Cambridge University Press.

Deci, E. L., Kasser, T., & Ryan, R. M. (1997). Self-determined teaching: Opportunities and obstacles. In J. L. Bess (Ed.), *Teaching well and liking it: Motivating faculty to teach effectively* (pp. 57-71). Baltimore, MD: Johns Hopkins University Press.

Deci, E. L., Eghrari, H., Patrick, B. C., & Leone, D. R. (1994). Facilitating internalization: The self-determination theory perspective. *Journal of Personality, 62*(1), 119.

Deci, E. L., & Ryan, R. M. (1985). *Intrinsic motivation and self-determination in human behavior*. New York: Plenum Press.

Deci, E. L., & Ryan, R. M. (2002). *Handbook of self-determination research*. Rochester, NY: University of Rochester Press.

Deci, E. L., Ryan, R. M., & Williams, G. C. (1996). Need satisfaction and the self-regulation of learning. *Learning and individual differences*, (8), 19.

Deci, E. L., Schwartz, A. J., Sheinman, L., & Ryan, R. M. (1981). An instrument to assess adults' orientations toward control versus autonomy with children: Reflections on intrinsic motivation and perceived competence. *Journal of Educational Psychology, 73*(5), 642-650.

Domitrovich, C. E., & Greenberg, M. T. (2000). The study of implementation: Current findings from effective programs that prevent mental disorders in school-aged children. *Journal of Educational and Psychological Consultation, 11*, 193-221.

Dusenbury, L., Brannigan, R., Falco, M., & Hansen, W. B. (2003). A review of research on fidelity of implementation: Implications for drug abuse prevention in school settings. *Health Education Research, 18*, 237-256.

Ellis, G., Voelkl, J., & Morris, C. (1994). Measurement and analysis issues with explanation of variance in daily experience using the flow model. *Journal of Leisure Research, 26*, 337-356.

Garbarino, J. (1975). The impact of anticipated reward upon cross-age tutoring. *Journal of Personality and Social Psychology, 32*, 421-428.

Grolnick, W. S., & Ryan, R. M. (1987). Autonomy in children's learning: An experimental and individual difference investigation. *Journal of Personality and Social Psychology, 52*(5), 890-898.

Hill, E., & Sibthorp, J. (2006). Autonomy support at diabetes camp: A self determination theory approach to therapeutic recreation. *Therapeutic Recreation Journal, 40*(2), 107-125.

Iso-Ahola, S. E. (1980). *The social psychology of leisure and recreation.* Dubuque, IA: William C. Brown.

Kahn, P. H. Jr. (1999). *The human relationship with nature.* Cambridge, MA: MIT Press.

Kaplan, R., Kaplan, S., & Ryan, R. L. (1998). *With people in mind: design and management for everyday nature.* Washington, D.C.: Island Press.

Kasser, T., & Ryan, R. M. (1993). A dark side of the American dream: Correlates of intrinsic and extrinsic goals. *Personality and Social Psychology Bulletin, 22,* 280-287.

Kasser, T., & Ryan, R. M. (2001). Further examining the American dream: differential correlates of intrinsic and extrinsic goals. In P. Schmuck & K.M Sheldon (Eds.), *Life goals and well-being: Toward a positive psychology of human striving.* Seattle, WA: Hogrefe & Huger.

Koestner, R. Ryan, R. M., Bernieri, F., & Holt, K. (1984). Setting limits on children's behavior: The differential effects of controlling versus informational styles on intrinsic motivation and creativity. *Journal of Personality, 52,* 233-248.

Legault, L., & Pelletier, L. G. (2000). Assessment of an educational environmental program's impact on students' and their parents' attitudes motivation, and behaviors. *Canadian Journal of Behavioral Science,* 32, 243-250.

Long, T., Ellis, G., Trunnell, E., Tatsugawa, K., & Freeman, P. (2001). Animating recreation experiences through the COMPLEX model. *Journal of Park and Recreation Administration, 2,* 1-22.

Mannell, R. C. (1989). *Leisure satisfaction.* In E. L. Jackson, & T. L. Burton (1989). *Understanding leisure and recreation: mapping the past and charting the future* (pp. 281-301). State College, PA: Venture.

Moore, R. C. (1997). The need for nature: A childhood right. *Social Justice,* 24, 203.

Nix, G. A., Ryan, R. M., Manly, J. B., & Deci, E. L. (1999). Revitalization through self-regulation: The effects of autonomous and controlled motivation on happiness and vitality. *Journal of Experimental Social Psychology, 35,* 266-284.

Nussbaum, M. C. (2001). *Upheavals of Thought: The Intelligence of Emotions.* Cambridge: Cambridge University Press.

Ortony, A., Clore, G. L., & Collins, A. (1988). *The cognitive structure of emotions.* Cambridge, MA: Cambridge University Press.

Osgood, C. E., Suci, G. J., & Tannenbaum, P. H. (1957). *The measurement of meaning.* Urbana: University of Illinois Press.

Patrick B. C., Skinner, E. A., & Connell, J. P. (1993). What motivates children's behavior and emotion? Joint effects of perceived control and autonomy in the academic domain. *Journal of Personality and Social Psychology, 65,* 781-791.

Pine, J. B., & Gilmore, J. H. (1999). *The experience economy: Work is theatre and every business a stage.* Boston: Harvard Business School Press.

Ralston, L., Ellis, G., Compton, D., & Lee, J.-W. (2006). *Staging memorable events and festivals: An integrated model of service and experience factors.* Paper presented at the Gobal Events Congress, Brisbane, Australia.

Pyzdek, T. (2003). *The Six Sigma handbook.* New York: McGraw-Hill.

Ramsing, R. (2005). *Predictors of autonomy support at diabetes summer camp: A self-determination theory approach.* Unpublished Dissertation, University of Utah, Salt Lake City.

Roark, M., & Ellis, G. (2007). Effect of staging strategies on situational self-determination among adolescent participants in a resident camp recreation activity. Paper presented at the *Third International Self-Determination Theory Conference.* Toronto, CA, May 25-27, 2007.

Radenbush, S. W., & Bryk, A. S. (2002). *Hierarchical linear models: applications and data analysis methods* (2nd ed.). Thousand Oaks, CA: Sage.

Reeve, J. (2005). *Understanding motivation and emotion* (4th ed.). Hoboken, NJ: John Wiley & Sons.

Reeve, J., Bolt, E., & Cai, Y. (1999). Autonomy-supportive teachers: How they teach and motivate students. *Journal of Educational Psychology, 91*(3), 537.

Rossman, J. R., & Schlatter, B. E. (2000). *Recreation programming: designing leisure experiences* (3rd ed.). Champaign, IL: Sagamore Publishing.

Ryan, R. M., & Deci, E. L. (2000). Self-determination theory and the facilitation of intrinsic motivation, social development, and well-being. *American Psychologist, 55*(1), 68.

Ryan, R. M., & Frederick, C. M. (1997). On energy, personality and health: Subjective vitality as a dynamic reflection of well-being. *Journal of Personality, 65*, 529-565.

Sheldon, K. M., Ryan, R. M., & Reis, H. T. (1996). What makes for a good day? Competence and autonomy in the day and in the person. *Personality and Social Psychology Bulletin, 22*, 1270-1279.

Skinner, E. (2002). Self-determination, coping, and development. In E. Deci & R. Ryan (Eds.), *Handbook of self-determination research* (pp. 297-337). Rochester, NY: The University of Rochester Press.

Solomon, R. C. (1988). On emotions as judgments. *American Philosophical Quarterly, 25*(2), 183-191.

Taylor, A. F., Kuo, F. E., & Sullivan, W. C. (2001). Coping with ADD: The surprising connection to green play settings. *Environment and Behavior, 33*, 54-77.

Taylor, A. F., Kuo, F. E., & Sullivan, W. C. (2002). Views of nature and self-discipline: Evidence from inner city children. *Journal of Environmental Psychology, 22*(1-2), pp. 49-63.

Walden, D. (Ed.). A special issue on Kano's methods for understanding customer-defined quality. *Center for Quality Management Journal, 2*(4), 2-36.

Wellborn, J. G. (1991). *Engaged and disaffected action: the conceptualization and measurement of motivation in the academic domain.* Unpublished doctoral dissertation, University of Rochester.

Wells, N., & Evans, G. (2003). Nearby nature: A buffer of life stress among rural children. *Environment and Behavior, 35*, 311-330.

Wilson, E. O. (1984). *Biophilia.* Cambridge, MA: Harvard University Press.

Wohlwill, J. F. (1974). Human adaptation to levels of environmental stimulation. *Human Ecology, 2*, 127-147.

Dialectical Behavioral Therapy and EMDR for Adolescents in Residential Treatment: A Practical and Theoretical Perspective

Carole Lovelle, PsyD, LCSW

INTRODUCTION

Adolescents who enter residential facilities often do so following and experience or series of experiences that are outside of the norm for others their age. Often, those experiences include traumatic events that have altered both their perceptions of the world and perhaps even their internal biochemical reactions (Bradley, 2003; Goleman, 1978; Gunnar & Barr, 1998; Kiraly, Ancill, & Dimitrovaand, 1997; Obrien, 1997; Sapolsky, 1994). They are then retraumatized as a result of suddenly and forcibly removed from their usual environment and away from their natural support systems. Trauma research clearly indicates that secondary wounding (retraumatization) may leave victims with more long-term damage than the original traumatic experience (Bloom, Bennington-Davis, Farragher; McCorkle, Nice-Martini, & Wellbank, Summer, 2003; Bloom & Reichert, 1998; Lalemand, Winter, 2005). The intensity of pathology is varied, the length of stay in these facilities is uncertain; thus, the need for immediate and effective treatment is imperative.

Recent focus on evidence-based practice coupled with active dissemination of research results has lead to the development of a number of interventions either strongly supported by empirical research or seen as promising due to the initial results of a limited number of studies. Five of these promising treatments are described in the Child Welfare League of America's Winter, 2007 edition of Focal Point. These treatments include: Adapted Cognitive-Behavioral Therapy Models for Physical and Sexual Abuse, Parent-Child Interaction Therapy, Child-Parent Psychotherapy for Family Violence, Cognitive-Behavioral Intervention for Children in Schools, and Project 12-Way/Safe Care for Child Neglect. All these methods use cognitive-behavioral interventions such as psychoeducation, skills training, and direct alteration of dysfunctional cognitions (Stambaugh, Burns, Landsverk, & Rolls Reutz, (Winder, 2007).

Substantial evidence also exists that trauma can produce physiological changes in survivors that may or may not be permanent. These changes place survivors in vulnerable chemical and psychological states in which they are particularly vulnerable to severe depression, anxiety, panic attacks, flashbacks, and other psyhcological disorders. Additional traumatic experiences, such as removal from a home, incarceration, and mistreatment within a facility, can worsen these conditions. It is therefore, essential that children and adolescents in state custody be: (1) removed from homes or residents in as gentle and humane a manner as possible, (2) housed in environments that are safe and well-managed, and (3) provided with treatment that is both sensitive and effective. This article addresses the third item: that treatment of trauma survivors in child and adolescent residential treatment be both sensitive and effective.

TRAUMA IN ADOLESCENTS

The study of the effects of trauma on the human psyche became serious during the Viet Nam War. Early work was done to assist the soldiers in recovering from the horrible memories of war so they could reenter society successfully. The effects of traumatic experiences were found to be so life encompassing that victims of domestic violence, victims and witnesses of violent crime were added to the studies of trauma treatment. Victims of child abuse and neglect were later added to studies of the effects of trauma (Shapiro, 2001).

On the psychological and mental levels, trauma refers to the wounding of the spirit, the emotions, the will to live, beliefs about the self and the world, one's sense of security. Trauma always involves a sense of helplessness or powerlessness in the victim. Trauma carries an element of entrapment, and a loss of the sense of safety and trust.

Post Traumatic Stress Disorder and Acute Stress disorder are the only diagnoses that place the origin of the symptoms on external events rather than on individual personality. These two diagnoses are the only ones to recognize that, subject to enough stress, any human being has the potential for developing stress symptoms and if the symptoms persist more than four weeks, PTSD or PTSD symptoms.

Over and over it has been concluded that the development of PTSD symptoms and the severity of these symptoms, has more to do with the intensity and duration of the symptoms than any preexisting personality patterns. This means that although the "pretrauma" personality, belief system and values do affect reactions to and interpretations of the traumatic event, PTSD does not develop because of some inherent weakness or inferiority in the personality. Trauma changes personalities, not the other way around. Study after study shows that when the stressor is sufficiently great, almost anyone can develop PTSD. The impact varies based on the duration, intensity, and the history of the person being traumatized (Figley, 1978; Kadushin, Boulanger, & Martin, 1981; Laufer, Yager, Frey-Wouters, & Donnellan, 1981; Shapiro, 2001).

Adolescents who enter residential facilities often express feeling weird, crazy, and somehow different from their peers. This comes at a time in their lives when peer acceptance is most critical to their development. Therefore treatment for them must include acceptance, and normalization of the way they feel based on their history and circumstances.

Judith Lyons (1991) found that those who recover most quickly and thoroughly are those with the following advantages:

1. Good health that is not significantly impaired by the trauma
2. No physical disfigurement as a result of the trauma
3. Adequate financial support or services
4. The ability to resume functioning in some if not all of the pretrauma roles
5. A supportive network of significant others

Please note that adolescents in a residential facility generally do not have their own money and many do not receive adequate and timely services. If we assume that part of the trauma resulted as a result of removal from their home or multiple failed foster families, they are able to assume few of their pretrauma roles. They are frequently denied access to a normal support system. The sense of helplessness is great for these individuals.

The Biochemistry of Trauma

Adolescents struggle with self-esteem issues. Society, friends or family may further damage the self-esteem because living in a residential facility may cause unjust stigmatization. As a result they may learn to numb out of dissociate from their most painful emotions. They may also overreact to situations, feel panic or become hypervigilant. They often want to change this but feel powerless to do so. The powerlessness experienced with regard to their emotional responses and behavior only reinforces the powerlessness experienced during the original traumatic event. This is referred to as secondary wounding and can actually have deeper and more long lasting effects than the original trauma.

Therapy that provides adolescents with information that this power-lessness may be out of their control is indicated. They need to know that overreacting or under reacting to situations may be biochemically deter-mined. Teachers, caregivers, and therapists as well as the adolescent need to know that controlling the experience of heightened anxiety, or feelings of rage may be automatic responses. They may be good at tun-ing out reactions appropriate to traumatic situations, but not to normal life events. Adrenaline increases can lead to a fight of flight or a freeze reaction as well as to biochemical shifts in certain neurotransmitters Since these neurotransmitters are involved in regulating emotions, changes in their function can have serious consequences for the survi-vor's ability to handle subsequent intense emotional experiences and life stresses.

The adrenal glands are highly reactive to life threatening to situations. They secrete large doses of adrenaline or noradrenalin in response to the threat of danger. Adrenaline provides a super charge of energy, which en-ables people to move with more energy and power than usual. The heart rate increases, pupils dilate, digestion slows down, and blood coagulates quicker. The lungs become more efficient, smells and other sensory data become sharper. In contrast, noradrenalin makes people freeze or go numb. As this happens, people become totally ineffective and may suffer intense guilt later for what they are not able to do. Surges of increased adrenaline may cause a depletion of neurotransmitters, the primary method of modu-lating emotions (Matsakis, 1991). Adolescents often feel less "like a freak" when they understand that their emotional and physical responses may, in fact, be out of their control.

Trauma as a Diagnosis

The simple definition of trauma is the impact on the organism of a traumatic event. This approach to trauma is imbedded in the DSM IV TR criteria for posttraumatic stress disorder (PTSD), which require the presence of a traumatic event. The traumatic event is described in the DSM IV TR as including two features:

1. The person experienced, witnessed or was confronted with an event or events that involved actual or threatened death or serious injury, or a threat to the physical integrity of the self or others.
2. The person's response involved intense fear, helplessness or horror. (In younger people this may be expressed as agitated or disorganized behavior.)

Certain events are so egregious that they are commonly acknowledged as traumatic. Some of these might include the removal of a child from her home for the first time, a series of failed foster home placements, witnessing the death or injury of a parent, and the repeated ineffectiveness of parental care over time. Most children coming into residential care have experienced more than one traumatic event in their lives. It is the errors of omission by the parents, not the errors of commission, which are the fundamental problems. The deeper trauma is the absence of love, affection, care and protection. The trauma is not being special to mom and dad.

Such trauma does not meet the first criteria for PTSD, but indeed represents a deeper, longer lasting trauma. To the trauma clinician, it is trauma to the person's attachment systems during childhood that counts. The betrayal of trust is often more hurtful than the abusive event. Childhood incest and emotional neglect are surely traumatic, but do not meet criteria A for PTSD if they are not accompanied by threats of violence, or if there is no threat of malnourishment.

In working with adolescents in a treatment facility trauma is defined as a complex interaction of external events and the individual's response to them. In parsing the domain of maladaptive behavior in children and adolescents, the field has made a fundamental distinction between:

1. Disruptive or externalizing behavior problems which include aggressive, antisocial, hyperactive, impulsive and sometimes inattentive behaviors, and
2. Internalizing problems (formerly emotional or over controlled problems), which include somatic complaints, social withdrawal, dysphoric affect, anxiety, and thought disturbance.

These two "broad band" domains that have been documented from the early days of empirical research in the field (e.g., Jenkins and Glickman,

1947; Peterson 1961) yield orthogonal dimensions in factor analysis study and form the basis for much current conceptualization about child and adolescent psychology (e.g., Quay, 1986).

It has become quite clear though that there is marked overlap exists between disruptive and internalizing problems (Achenbach 1991a, 1991b; Biederman, Newcorn, & Sprich 1991). Diagnostic comorbidity is of extreme importance in treatment planning (Shaffer, p. 92), These studies form the basis for much of the current research of child pathology (Shaffer, p. 92). Both DBT and EMDR are effective in a milieu setting with adolescents experiencing this overlap.

OVERVIEWS OF DBT AND EMDR

Both DBT and EMDR use processes that are grounded in cognitive-behavioral techniques. DBT focuses on such skills and behaviors as mindfulness and distress management. During these processes survivors are taught new behavioral alternatives to replace their old, trauma-induced behavioral repertoires. They also address dysfunctional cognitions that have kept them tied to old behaviors. EMDR uses intentional exposure to thoughts about traumatic incidents, while employing planned eye movement and sometimes tactile and auditory experiences to reintegrate brain activity.

Processes and Techniques in DBT

Marcia Linehan's (1993) Dialectical Behavior Therapy (DBT) is a wonderfully effective treatment that can be adapted to a variety of settings. It was originally developed for use with patients experiencing Borderline Personality Disorder. However, the strategies and techniques she outlined have robust applicability beyond borderline personality disorder. In fact, Dr. Linehan has outlined an eclectic treatment approach that is especially powerful with patients who have mood, anxiety, addictive, eating, impulse-control and personality disorders.

Since training with Linehan in 1994 at the Menninger clinic, the current author has used the techniques with many patients meeting criteria for many other diagnoses. Currently, the techniques are used in individual treatment with adolescent boys who are in state's custody and live in a residential facility. Both individual and group treatment is provided for girls in states custody who reside at another facility. DBT is effective from the first day of treatment for these teen-agers. Results have been best when DBT begins in the first individual session, then is carried over into traditional DBT groups using Linehan's (1993) workbook, *Skills Training for Treating Borderline Personality Disorder.* Alterations in the format for use with younger clients are minimal and the workbook provides effective tools for working with traumatized teen-agers. While these youngsters feel powerless, it is good to have care-givers who listen and accept their stories and their feelings as valid for their situation.

DBT addresses the core issue of emotional dysregulation. Teen-agers who suffer intense emotional pain frequently engage in emotional avoidance and escape behaviors. They do not want to feel what they feel. Therefore, they attempt to truncate those feelings to what they perceive are more manageable levels. In so doing they are likely to engage in destructive and potentially self-harming behaviors.

Like psychodynamic approaches DBT assumes that repression of affect is central to emotional pathology. Adolescents who reside in a group facility with non-family members have difficulty expressing several if not all emotions. Prolonged intensity of affect results in high baseline arousal even in non-threatening environments. Group residential facilities can be extremely threatening especially when the adolescent is there as a result of attempting to escape what he/she feels.

DBT assumes that the intensity of affect is caused by dialectic conflict between the self and the environment. This can generate inadequate compromises between competing needs and wants including attachment, trauma and loss experiences and genetic or kindling effects. The conflicts between the adolescent and his residential facility include numerous possibilities. Some of those possibilities are illustrated in Table 1 below.

Emotional dysregulation is viewed as a joint outcome of biological disposition, environmental context and the transaction between the two during development. This may be described to adolescents as being born with intense and unusual emotional sensitivity and spending time in an invalidating environment.

TABLE 1. Typical Conflicts of Adolescence

I'm fragile and I'll get hurt if I get close to someone	⟺	I'm extremely lonely
People will see my deficiencies If I get close enough	⟺	Better to be alone Than to feel bad
It is shameful that I feel so deeply	⟺	I must hide my sensitivity from others
I'm socially empty I have nothing to say	⟺	I need to talk
I'm not hurt	⟺	You are ruining my life
I am superior To most people	⟺	I do not fit in anywhere
I hate this place	⟺	I have nowhere to go
I hate you	⟺	Please don't Leave me
I love you	⟺	I never want to see you again

DBT accepts the bio-physiological aspects of trauma and one core assumption is that there is a function for every behavior and attitude no matter how irrational or self-harming it may appear to be. The most damaging invalidation finds its origin in the home. By the time the child enters the residential facility this may have been intensified by school failures, bulling, peer pressure, substance abuse and/or the court system. This creates the secondary wounding that drives the wound even deeper. The intensity and duration of the trauma, and the secondary wounding experiences combined with the genetic make-up of the adolescent create physiological damage. This can make the teen-ager's responses automatic and often out of their control.

DBT accepts the patients' core belief about themselves as valid for the experience they have. DBT therapy also accepts the patients' view of the problems as exactly the way it is for them. This includes the present as well as their account of history. Teen-agers relate to therapists and other professionals that listen and accept what they say as valid. This is especially powerful in a group setting. Adolescents respond more honestly with peer support.

DBT deals with emotions first and suggests that the patient's thoughts are normal based on what they have experienced. DBT finds it invalidating to imply that the patient's thoughts are distorted. Cognitive therapy is introduced later when emotions are calm and trust is established with the therapist.

DBT therapists recognize and validate every effort the patient uses to calm the chaos in his/her life. Therapists accept what is now, while teaching the patient more effective skills. The therapist openly acknowledges that the patient's efforts and actions have allowed him to survive until this time and does not seek to strip away old coping methods (unless they involve suicidal or other high risk behaviors), until more effective skills are incorporated into their behavior.

This is accomplished through well-defined skill development following a prescribed course of treatment. These skills may be learned in individual or group settings. In adolescent residential facilities, skills training within a group setting works best, while using EMDR and other types of therapy in individual sessions.

Seasoned professionals, Linehan and Marra each have detailed plans for conducting DBT groups. (For specific plans that may be copied with both of the authors' permission see the reference page of this article.) The writer uses a combination of these two plans along with EMDR and adjunct therapies, and materials gathered while facilitating 25 DBT groups of 32 weeks over the past 13 years.

If emotional arousal is defined not just as mental and physical symptoms of anxiety, but also as depressed affect, negative appraisals, anticipation of danger and threat, excitability or the lack or it, and general existential disease, then most mental disorders are appropriate for DBT treatment. The DBT modules include: (1) Meaning Making, 6 weeks duration, (2) Mindfulness, 6-8 weeks duration, (3) Interpersonal Relationship Skills, 2-4 weeks duration, (4) Emotional Regulation Skills, 6-8 weeks duration, (5) Distress Tolerance, 2-4 week's duration, and (6) Strategic Behavior (unspecified duration). The modules are clearly described and techniques to be used for each are described in the treatment manuals of both Linehan and Marra.

Processes and Techniques in EMDR

EMDR is also widely used to treat persons who have experienced trauma. While EMDR greatly assists the patient to reduce the devastating impact of painful memories of traumatic events, it does little to provide compassionate warmth and acceptance or to teach them the skills necessary to live their lives with less emotional chaos and increased effectiveness.

EMDR is based on the work of Shapiro (1995), who proposed the accelerated information processing theory. This concept is consistent with extant trauma processing theories to account for the effects seen with EMDR. According to accelerated information processing, humans are designed to heal naturally from emotional wounds, just as they are from physical wounds. Healing involves a process of progressive integration of the upsetting memory aspects, through activities such as talking, thinking, feeling and dreaming until the memory is completely worked through. The memory becomes neutralized. However, when the memory is so overwhelming that it shocks the system, the healing process may be blocked and the disturbing information does not get integrated. Disturbing aspects of the memory is locked in raw, unprocessed form and disturbing features of the memory may emerge as posttraumatic symptoms (Greenwald, p. 120). The role of EMDR is to help the client access and metabolize the memory, and transform it to a more neutral and healthier form. EMDR is distinguished from other trauma treatments by the accelerated information processing effect, which in most cases condenses the healing process into a very brief period.

The EMDR protocol is designed to access and reprocess all the elements of a traumatic memory. The protocol includes a number of component tools that assist in focusing on the memory, facilitating reprocessing and tracking. It is important for the clinician to be sensitive to the client's feelings. This is especially true with adolescents. They must not be frustrated for not giving "the right answers." Plain language should always be used when dealing with adolescents. The clinician should always be quick to take the blame for any misunderstanding: "I guess I didn't explain that right." EMDR is rarely used alone as a therapeutic technique. It is used well with cognitive therapy, traditional psychotherapy, Gestalt, and DBT. The standard protocol of EMDR in combination with DBT is as follows:

1. Phase one: Taking a complete client history, including client readiness, safety factors and dissociation screening. Targets are addressed to include past, present and future. With DBT a complete history is taken, including medical, social and family history, client's present environment, medical and substance abuse history, and thoughts about the future.
2. Phase two: Preparation, creating a bond with the client, setting expectations, creating a safe place and testing the eye movements or Dual Attention Stimulus (DAS). DBT does much the same with the exception of the use of DAS.
3. Phase three: Assessment includes selecting the picture that represents the target. DBT also accepts the view of the client's problem as the problem; identifying a negative core belief (NC), DBT identifies the self concept of the patient as a target for therapy; developing a positive cognition (PC), DBT assists the patient to set positive therapeutic goals: rating the validity of the positive cognition (VOC), DBT assesses the confidence level of the patient and validates previous efforts at recovery while identifying conflicts and barriers to the success of treatment; naming the emotion, DBT assists in helping the patient to calm emotional chaos; estimates the subjective units of disturbance (SUDS), assesses the numerical value of each symptom on a scale of 1-10; and identifying

body sensations, DBT also gets this information in the assessment phase of treatment.

4. Phase four: Desensitization includes reprocessing the memory using DAS, according to standard protocols, DBT therapists add validation to the patient while processing the memory.
5. Phase five: Installing the positive cognition while holding the memory in mind, enhanced through validation.
6. Phase six: Body scan, searching for additional body sensations, DBT refers to this as mindfulness.
7. Phase seven: Closure, includes homework to monitor changes, expectations, and if needed, bringing the client to a state of equilibrium, DBT skills training is valuable to the client to assist in rebuilding their life after closure of EMDR.
8. Phase eight: Reevaluation, includes checking in at the next session to see if the client requires new processing for the previous target or associated material, DBT picks up to continue to validate progress, identify continuing conflicts and teach useful life skills.

THE "FIT" OF DBT AND EMDR WITH RESIDENTIAL TREATMENT

DBT and EMDR are an excellent fit for the residential setting. Where staff are trained in either or both staff can provide the treatment. Where staff do not have the necessary training, facilities can contract with outside providers to provide the services. In many settings it may be more practical to utilize a mixture of staff and contract therapists. For example, staff might provide individual counseling while outside therapists lead groups and offer EMDR. In DBT there is strong collaboration between individual therapists and group therapists. Observations from sessions are shared as necessary. Individual therapists review homework assigned in group with clients to gain insight into client needs and progress. In such an arrangement periodic group staffings might be useful. Certainly, a reliable system of regular communication and exchange of documents would need to be established.

Length of participation might be an issue with some juveniles. Although EMDR is a short-term treatment, DBT continues over a period of months. Early graduation, elopement from treatment, and state-authorized relocations could bring juveniles' participation to an early end.

Most of these situations can be planned for, leading the departing youth and the other group members through a termination process (for the departing member) over the remaining time in treatment. If departure is scheduled abruptly, a special meeting could easily be arranged. Materials for additional study could be provided to the departing juvenile and arrangements made to continue the treatment elsewhere. Elopements should be handled directly and honestly, so that there is no doubt as to why a juvenile suddenly stops attending group sessions. Should a youth return to the facility at a later time it will be necessary for to complete missed homework assignments.

As when any trauma work is conducted, staff should be prepared to deal with youths' mood swings, outbursts, flashbacks, and other experiences related to their history of trauma. In fact, the residential aspect of the proposed treatment makes it in many ways ideal for dealing with these kinds of situations. Juveniles would have immediate access to competent help should the need for that help arise.

DOCUMENTED OUTCOMES FOR DBT AND EMDR

The current author has reported her own successful experiences as well as those of her colleagues in using both DBT and EMDR with adolescents who have experienced severe trauma. There is also a substantial body of empirical literature supporting the use of both modalities for adults with a number of different conditions.

Outcomes for DBT

DBT has been found to be effective for an assortment of conditions including borderline personality disorder (Linehan et al., 1991; Verheul et al., 2003) depression (Bohus et al., 2000; Bradley & Fallingstad, 2003), suicidal ideation (Bohus et al., 2000), dissociation (Bohus et al., 2000), stress (Bohus et al., 2000), self-harm (Bohus et al., 2000; Hawton et al., 2000) , substance abuse (Linehan et al., 1991; Linehan et al., 1999), and eating disorders (Telch, Agas, & Linehan, 2001). These same studies have found DBT to be effective across multiple treatment settings from private practice to residential programs, and across multiple age groups, from adolescents to elders. The current author has also used it successfully with person with bipolar disorder, dissociative disorders, and persons with psychotic disorders.

Outcomes for EMDR

EMDR has also received extensive clinical testing and has been supported in numerous trials as effective for treating trauma and trauma-related disorders. Sixteen randomized trials and 6 non-randomized trials have found EMDR to be superior to other forms of therapy for treating trauma. A single, non-randomized trial found cognitive behavior therapy to be more effective than DBT (EMDR Institute, 2007). In addition, a meta-analysis conducted by Van Etten and Taylor (1998) concluded that EMDR and behavior therapy were both more effective than psychotropic medication.

It is important to recall that, in successfully treating trauma-related disorders, several other conditions may be alleviated. For example, anxiety and depression may be reduced or the tendency to dissociate may be lessened. EMDR has not been tested and is not recommended for many disorders, yet some of the effects and conditions found in those disorders may be improved or eliminated if they are the result of trauma.

CONCLUSION

Both DBT and EMDR are effective, evidence-based approaches to treating conditions produced by trauma, such as post-traumatic stress disorder. They are based on sound theory and are consistent with both other well-supported and with what has been learned through empirical tests of other treatment methods. Both have been shown to be effective in clinical trials. DBT is effective for treating additional conditions that may exist comorbidly with or be related to stress disorders. The current author has used them conjointly to produce positive benefits in a variety of age groups. DBT and EMDR, administered conjointly, remain a little-explored, yet highly promising approach to providing sensitive, effective residential treatment for adolescents.

REFERENCES

Achenbach, T.M. (1966). The Classification of Children's psychiatric symptoms: A factor-analytic study. Psychological Monographs 80, Whole number 615.

Bloom, S.L., Bennington-Davis, M., Farragher, B., McCorkle, D., Nice-Martini, K., Bloom, S.L., & Reichert, M. (1998). *Bearing witness: Trauma and collective responsibility.* Binghamton, NY: Haworth Press.

Bohus, M., Haaf, B., Striglmayr, C., Pohl, U., Bohme, R., & Linehan, M.M. (2000). Evaluation of inpatient dialectical behavioral therapy for borderline personality disorder–a prospective study. *Behavior Research and Therapy, 38(9),* 875-887.

Bradley, S.J. (2000). *Affect regulation and the development of psychopathology.* New York: Guilford Press.

Bradley, R.G., & Fallingstad, D.R. (2003). Group therapy for incarcerated women who experienced interpersonal violence: A pilot study. *Journal of Traumatic Stress, 16(4),* 337-340.

EMDR Institute. (2007). Efficacy of EMDR. (Available online: http://www.emdr.com/efficacy.htm).

Figley, C.R. (1978). Psychosocial adjustment among Vietnam veterans:. In C.R. Figley (Ed.), Stress disorders among Vietnam veterans: Theory, research, and treatment. New York: Brunner/Mazel.

Goleman, D. (2003). A taxonomy of meditation-specific altered states. *Journal of Altered States of Consiousness, 4(2),* 203-213.

Greenwald, R. (1994). Applying eye movement desensitization and reprocessing (EMDR) to the treatment of traumatized children: Five case studies. *Anxiety Disorders Practice Journal, 1,* 83-97.

Gunnar, M.R., & Barr, R.G. (1998). Stress, early brain development, and behavior. *Infants and Young Children, 11,* 1-14.

Hawton, K., Townsend, E., Arensmann, E., Gunnel, D., Hazell, P., & House, A. (2000). Psychosocial versus pharmacological treatments for deliberate self-harm. *Cochrane Database Syst Rev, (2),* CD001764.

Kadushin, C., Boulanger, G., & Martin, J. (1981). Long-term stress reactions : Some causes, consequences, and naturally-occurring support systems. In A. Egendorf, C. Kadushin, P.S. Laufer, G. Rothbart, & L. Sloan (Eds.) *Legacies of Vietnam: Comparative adjustment of veterans and their peers.* New York: Center for Policy Research.

Kiraly, S., Ancill, R.J., & Dimitrova, G. (1997). The relationship of endogenous cortisol to psychiatric disorder: A review. *Canadian Journal of Psychiatry, 42,* 415-420.

Lalemand, K. (Winter, 2005). Residential child care: Guidelines for physical techniques, crisis prevention, and management. *Child Welfare League of America Residential Treatment Quarterly, (5)3,* 5-7.

Laufer, R.S., Yager, T., Frey-Wouters, E., & Donnellan, J. (1981). Post-war trauma: Social and psychological problems of Vietnam veterans in the aftermath of the Vietnam War. In A. Egendorf, C. Kadushin, P.S. Laufer, G. Rothbart, & L. Sloan (Eds.) *Legacies of Vietnam: Comparative adjustment of veterans and their peers.* New York: Center for Policy Research.

Linehan, M.M. (1993). *Skills training for treating borderline personality disorder.* New York: The Guilford Press.

Linehan, MM., Armstrong, H.E., Suarez, A., Allmon, D., & Heard, H.L. (1991). Dialectical behavioral therapy versus comprehensive validation therapy plus 12-step for the treatment of opioid dependent women meeting criteria for borderline personality disorder. *Drug and alcohol dependence, 67(1),* 13-26.

Linehan, M.M., Schmidt, H., III, Dimeff, L.A., Craft, J.C., Kanter, J., & Comtois, K.A. (1999). Dialectical behavior therapy for patients with borderline personality disorder and drug-dependence. *American Journal of Addictions, 8(4),* 279-292.

Marra, T. (2005). *Dialectical behavior therapy in private practice: A practical and comprehensive guide.* Oakland, CA: New Harbinger Publications.

Matsakis, A. (1991). *I can't get over it: A handbook for trauma survivors.* Oakland, CA: New Harbinger Publications.

Obrien, J.T. (1997). The 'glucocorticol cascade hypothesis': Prolonged stress may cause permanent brain damage. *British Journal of Psychiatry, 170,* 199-201.

Sapolsky, R.M. (1994). *Why zebras don't get ulcers: A guide to stress, stress-related disorders, and coping.* New York: Freeman.

Shaffer, D. (1984). The clinical guide to child psychology. New York: Free Press.

Shapiro, F. (2001). *Eye movement desensitization and reprocessing.* New York: The Guilford Press.

Telch, C.F., Agras, W.S., & Linehan, M.M. (2001). Dialectic behavior therapy for binge eating disorder. *Journal of Counseling and Clinical Psychology, 69(6),* 1061-1065.

Van Etten, M., & Taylor, S. (1998). Comparative efficacy of treatment for post-traumatic stress disorder: A meta-analysis. *Clinical Psychology and Psychotherapy, 5,* 126-144.

Verheul, R., Van Den Bosch, L.M., Koeter, M.W., De Ridder, M.A., Stijnen, T., & Van Den Brink, W. (2003). Dialectical behavioral therapy for women with borderline personality disorder: 12 month, randomized clinical trial in the Netherlands. *British Journal of Psychiatry, 182,* 135-140.

Combining Drug Court
with Adolescent Residential Treatment:
Lessons from Juvenile and Adult Programs

Samuel A. MacMaster, PhD
Rodney A. Ellis, PhD, CMSW
Tammy Holmes, MA

INTRODUCTION

This paper combines an evaluation of a currently operating juvenile drug court in Middle Tennessee with recommendations for the inclusion of a residential component in juvenile drug courts. These recommendations are based in the experiences of a residential drug court program in Davidson County (Nashville), Tennessee. Interventions over the last several years have followed the early findings of Jessor and Jessor (1977), who identified substance abuse among juveniles as one of a cluster of several adolescent problem behaviors sharing a root cause. Perhaps the most visible example is the more recent work of Henggler (1999) whose Multi-Systemic Therapy (MST) has demonstrated remarkable results with juveniles who use substances was well as those who engage in other problem behaviors. These findings, however, may have produced a biased perspective from those who fund, develop, and evaluate programs for troubled juveniles. Despite excellent outcomes for many youth, substantial numbers remain for whom treatment is less than successful. Although it is unrealistic to anticipate success with all youth, it is apparent that some for whom current interventions are not effective might benefit from alternative forms of treatment.

One alternative that has proven successful for many different age groups is drug court. Although designating substance abuse as a target behavior is not consistent with a problem behavior approach, many of its philosophies as well many MST strategies have been incorporated into the intervention. Drug court as it exists today was established for adults. The first was founded 1989 by Janet Reno who was, at the time, State Attorney for the eleventh judicial circuit in Miami, FL (Belenko, S., 1998). Since that time courts have proliferated, in large part because of aggressive funding and training support from the federal government and the National Drug Court Institute (Roberts, Brophy, & Cooper, March, 1997). Writing at the end of 2004, Huddleston, Freeman-Wilson, Marlowe, and Roussell reported that 1,621 courts were operating worldwide, 357 of which were for juveniles.

Drug courts use a team approach which combines the power of the court with treatment. Participation is often voluntary, with offenders being able to avoid incarceration and perhaps have their records expunged if they are successful in their treatment. Team members from the court, the prosecutor's office, the public defender's office, probation, and treatment meet regularly review participants' progress. Typically, the team meets before a court session beings to discuss whatever cases may be on the docket for that session. All the program participants attend every session, regardless of whether their name is on the docket. A specified set of rewards and sanctions are used to encourage abstinence and prosocial behavior. Although abstinence is encouraged, the probability that "slips" will occur is acknowledged. Participants typically are not removed from the program the first or second time they use (Belenko, 1996; McPhail & McNulty, 1995; Cooper, May, 2001).

Juvenile drug courts provide intensive and authoritative supervision of juveniles who have come to the attention of the court due to substance-related delinquent or status offenses. At the same time, they provide coordinated, collaborative services to assist youths and their families in a number of area, including substance abuse, mental health counseling, family counseling, and educational support (Cooper, May, 2001). As the literature review and the data from the current study will show, they are effective for many juveniles. Some juveniles, however, are not as successful. There are sound reasons to believe that specific enhancements, such as the one recommended in this paper, would lead to success among larger numbers of juveniles. The purpose of this paper, then, is to present the results of an evaluation of a juvenile drug court, then to propose specific enhancements that might be made to improve outcomes in similar settings.

LITERATURE REVIEW

According to the National Drug Court Institute (NDCI) three general types of analyses of drug courts have been conducted. These types include process evaluations, cost savings analyses, and impact evaluations. The majority have been process evaluations, in which the operations of various courts have been monitored. They have helped NDCI identify key indicators, determine the degree to which the target population is being served, and understand more about the characteristics of the program participants (Belenko, 1998).

A few studies have tried to determine whether the cost savings that theoretically should be present with drug courts is indeed present. In fact, results have shown such courts to save substantially over conventional means of treatment. Drug courts are recognized as a cost-effective alternative to traditional methods of processing offenders (Belenko, 1998; Huddleson, Freeman-Wilson, Marlowe, & Roussell, 2005).

Several impact or outcome evaluations of drug courts have also been conducted. Although the percentages have varied, program effectiveness has often been supported. First, drug use has been substantially decreased for some participants while they were actually in the program. These results compared favorably to those for participants in other types of programs (Belenko, 1998; Huddleson, Freeman-Wilson, Marlowe, & Roussell, 2005; Rand Corporation, 1997; Terry III, 1998). Further, post-program recidivism rates have consistently been lower for drug court participants. They engage in consistently less criminal behavior and substance abuse then do those from other types of programs (Belenko, 1998; Finegan, 1996; Huddleson, Freeman-Wilson, Marlowe, & Roussell, 2005; Rempel et al., 2003).

Juvenile drug courts incorporate the same components as do adult courts, but have have some additional elements. According to Cooper (May, 2001), shared elements include:

1. A drug court team is assembled that includes judge, prosecutor, public defender, treatment provider(s), evaluator, and a representative of the school system.
2. First contact with the court is arranged as soon as possible after the offense and frequent contact is arranged with the judge. For example, many jurisdictions hold weekly, mandatory meetings for all drug court participants in the form of court sessions. Although all participants attend these sessions, only selected cases are on the docket for each session.

3. A comprehensive treatment plan is developed for each participant.
4. Services are provided and coordinated by the court and members of the treatment team.
5. Regular supervision and monitoring of participants is accomplished through drug screening, supervision, and case management.
6. Immediate response by the court to both progress and non-compliance on the part of participants.
7. A judge who is concerned about the well-being of participants, who is culturally sensitive, and who is familiar with the kinds of life processes experienced by participants (for example, for juveniles, the processes in adolescent development).
8. A focus on the strengths and abilities of participants.

Roberts, Brophy, and Cooper (1997) recommend the following enhancements for juvenile drug courts:

1. A comprehensive initial assessment followed by regular follow-up assessment throughout the program.
2. Integration of assessment information with all decisions made during the treatment process.
3. A focus on family relationships and their impact on the participant.
4. Coordination of services by and between the court, treatment providers, the school system, and other community agencies.
5. Knowledge by the treatment team about processes of adolescent development and how those processes may related to substance abuse.

METHODOLOGY

The current study was conducted during a one year period at the Upper Cumberland Juvenile Drug Court in central Tennessee. Seven area counties have drug court programs: Putnam, White, Cumberland, Dekalb, Jackson, Pickett, and Overton. The courts are operated collaboratively, with members of the drug court teams sharing responsibilities across the jurisdiction. Although the area includes Cookville, a community of 26,000, designated as one of the country's micropolitan areas, it is predominantly rural. In fact, more than two thirds of the study's participants come from areas that are clearly identifiable as rural.

Sample and Data Collection

The sample consisted of all the participants in the juvenile drug court program between its inception in December, 2002 and May, 2007. Data were collected by the drug court coordinator with the assistance of court personnel in each jurisdiction.

Measurement

Three outcome variables were identified. The first, "arrests" was simply defined as any incident of new charges brought after a juvenile had entered the program. "Drug screens" referred to the results of a random urinalysis administered periodically by program personnel. Juveniles either tested "positive" indicating the presence of substances, or "negative" indicating the absence of those substances. "Family cohesion" was measured using the results of the Family Strengths Assessment administered at baseline and at the time of the program's completion.

Data Analysis

Data for the arrest and drug screen were analyzed by simple calculation of percentages. Data for family cohesion were analyzed using paired t-tests.

RESULTS

Sample Characteristics

One hundred and eighty-one individuals completed an initial interview and provided their own demographic information (see Table 1). Nearly all of the participants identified themselves as Caucasians (97.7%), and two-thirds (66.7%) were male. Average age of participant was 19.38 years at the time the study was conducted. For many this was nearly five years after they had received services. The court only accepts clients between the ages of 13 and 18. It is important to note current age because this speaks to the long-term effectiveness of the program. Low recidivism at higher ages would provide evidence of such effectiveness.

TABLE 1. Demographics

Demographic	Categories	Total Sample
Age (the figures in this category represent the ages of the participants at the time the study was conducted, not at the time services were actually received).	13-15 16-17 18-19 20-21 22	4 (2.2%) 32 (17.7%) 64 (35.5%) 68 (37.7%) 12 (6.7%)
Gender	Male Female	118 (66.7%) 59 (33.3%)
Ethnicity/Racial Background	Caucasian Hispanic/Latino Native American Other	177 (97.7%) 2 (1.1%) 1 (0.5%) 1 (0.5%)
Drug of Choice	Marijuana Alcohol Cocaine Methamphetamine Hallucinogens Heroin Inhalants Prescription Meds	28.1 23.4 10.5 7.7 5.8 4.9 4.9 0.9
County or Residence	Putnam White Cumberland Dekalb Jackson Pickett Overton Davidson Van Buren	50 38 36 32 8 8 7 1 1

Nearly three-fourths (73.2%) of respondents were between the ages of eighteen and twenty-one at the time of the study's preparation.

SERVICE UTILIZATION

Length of Service

Participants were involved in the program for an extended period of time. The average length of stay was 231 days, or nearly eight months. There was some variability in length of stay, as one individual stayed as few as twelve days and another stayed longer than two years (774 days).

Community Services Received

In addition to the drug court programming participants were referred to and received a wide variety of community services. Two hundred and forty-six services were provided consisting primarily of substance abuse related services. Services utilized by participants are presented in the table below.

Service Type	Specific Service	Participants Receiving Service
Substance Abuse	Substance Abuse Assessment	55
	Intensive Outpatient	39
	Alcohol and Drug Education	37
	Inpatient Treatment	31
	Residential Substance Abuse Treatment	6
Mental Health	Individual Counseling	20
	School-based Counseling	11
	Mental Health Counseling	6
	Anger Management	3
	Crisis Stabilization	3
	Psychiatric Services provided by MD	3
	Medication Management	2
	In-home Counseling	1
Other	Mentoring	11
	Community Health Services	4
	Family Preservation	3
	Parenting Counseling	2

Completion Rate

Of the one hundred and fifty-nine individuals who have been re-leased from the program, the majority (57.6%) successfully completed the program. Almost a quarter (23.8%) were placed in state custody, and a significant group (13.2%) were released for being non-compliant, and a small percentage (5.0%) moved out of the area before completing the program.

OUTCOMES

Arrests

One hundred and seventy individuals (93.9%) did not recidivate. However, eleven participants (6.1%) were rearrested after completing the program. There were a total of seventeen arrests. Five arrests for illegal consumption of alcohol, three arrests for possession of a controlled substance, two arrests for possession of drug paraphernalia, two arrests for burglary, and one arrest each for DUI, domestic abuse, and shoplifting. Two individuals were also arrested for failing to comply with the diversion program.

Drug Screens

Participants were often asked to submit to drug testing. The 181 participants had a total of 1,612 drug tests, an average of nearly nine tests per person. However there was a high degree of variability in the number of drug tests that individuals took, which ranged from as few as one to as many as forty-six tests. The vast majority of tests (98.9%) were urine drug screens, however participants also submitted to blood, hair follicle, and saliva tests. Substances were tested for alcohol, marijuana, cocaine, heroin, hallucinogens, nicotine, methamphetamines, and a panel of "other drugs."

Most tested samples (82.4%) did not test positive for any substance, and a small percentage were undetermined (1.2%). Samples that did test positive were most frequently positive for marijuana (13.0% of collected samples), cocaine (1.5%), methamphetamines (1.4%), alcohol (0.2%), and inhalants (0.1%). There were no positive tests for hallucinogens or heroin. Additionally, four percent of all of the samples tested positive for the other drug panel, these positive tests were primarily benzodiazepines.

Family Cohesion

The Family Strengths Assessment was used to measure changes between baseline and completion. For the 92 individuals who completed the program statistically significant differences were found on all subscales using paired samples t-tests. The results can be seen in the table below.

Subscale	Mean Difference	Significance
Household Community and Employment	2.31	.000
Mental Health	−3.10	.000
Medical	−3.63	.000
Legal	−1.92	.000
Education	−3.93	.001
Family-Child Interaction	−2.65	.000
Family-Caregiver Interaction	−4.52	.000
Social Support	−4.75	.000

DISCUSSION

The results of the study strongly support the effectiveness of the Putnam County Juvenile Drug court. Participants showed very low rates of arrest after completing the program. Drug screening was only done during the time youths were in the program, yet the very low rate of positive tests also supports program effectiveness. Also very telling were the results of the measure for family cohesion. Improvements were made across every area measured, suggesting that the court's approach was comprehensive and effective. Family cohesion is a strong protective factor against substance abuse and other problem behavior. The improvements on these scales indicate that the court was able not only to help juveniles refrain from problem behavior, but was also able to facilitate changes in their environments that can help them sustain their gains in the future.

LIMITATIONS

The study had a number of limitations. The sample size was small as compared to what I would have been in a large city over the same period of time. The small sample size and its relative homogeneity offer challenges to its generalizability. For example, although the more than 97% Caucasian sample is reflective of the demographics of the community, the study may offer limited insight in the degree to which the court would be effective for other ethnic groups. Similarly, given that the court only heard cases of juveniles between the ages of 14 to 18, the ability to generalize to younger children is also limited.

A second limitation has to do with the lack of a means of knowing whether youths began to use substances again after graduating from the program. No drug screening was done post-graduation. This limitation seems rather insignificant in the light of the very low recidivism rate also recorded. Although arrest for delinquent behavior cannot serve as a proxy for substance abuse, it could be considered informative. Given the history of this group of participants as well as the natural of adolescent problem behavior (Jessor and Jessor, 1979), the low number of delinquent offenses suggests a similarly low use of illicit substances.

One other limitation should be identified. The drug court coordinator was able to examine police and court records from the counties included in the study. This meant that any offenses committed within that area would have been identified. However, had offenses been committed in other areas they would not have been included in the data. The result may have been a very slight underreporting of delinquent offense.

RATIONALE FOR ADDING A RESIDENTIAL COMPONENT TO JUVENILE DRUG COURT

The Upper Cumberland Juvenile Drug Court and similar organizations around the country have supported as effective. Even the retention rates of many (the current study reported 56.7%) are well in excess of that identified by the Office of Applied Science (2007) as typical of most substance abuse treatment programs (about 40%). Still this means that almost 45% of the juveniles who enter treatment never complete it.

The inability of a substantial number of juveniles to complete programs suggests the importance of developing additional supervision and treatment alternatives. An example of such an alternative can be found in Davidson County (Nashville, TN).

The Davidson County Drug Court Residential Program

Davidson County, Tennessee is about an hour's drive west of Cookeville. It is home to the Davidson County Drug Court Residential Program (DC4), a long-term residential drug and alcohol treatment facility for adults. It is operated by employees of the Division IV Criminal Court in the 20th Judicial District. DC4 is believed to be the only self-operated residential drug court program in the country. The program is described on its Website at http://drugcourt.nashville.gov/portal/page/portal/drugCourt/home/.

The program has operated since 1997. Since that time 312 participants have graduated from the program. The completion rate has been excellent, approximately 65% as compared to an average of around 40% in typical drug treatment programs (OAS, 2007). The recidivism rate for successful completers has also been outstanding at approximately 25%. Many of the participants would be seen as particularly challenging at the time they enter the program. For example, most had 8 or more previous arrests, and many had been incarcerated for two to four years. Most were unemployed, lacking any stable job history. Program officials report that the average participant had been convicted of 5 prior non-violent felonies. Despite these challenges he court has maintained a negative drug test rate (for those in the program) of 97%, and a 100% employment rate for graduates.

Participants are referred to the program by a number of sources, for example, the public defenders office, private attorneys, or other local treatment programs. Upon referral participants meet with the Drug Court Assessment Team (similar in composition to the one in the Upper Cumberland Juvenile Drug Court), which determines whether they will receive intensive outpatient treatment and supervision of will be placed in the residential facility. A recommendation is then made to the court to admit the offender into the chosen program.

Participants are supervised by probation officers and receive a comprehensive assessment to identify chemical dependency, educational, employment, or medical needs. Based on the results of the assessment, a treatment plan is developed and services are put in place. Program goals include abstaining from addictive behaviors, abstaining from criminal behavior, gaining basic education and vocational training, and developing life skills such as anger management and communication skills.

The residential component of DC4 includes four phases: (1) assessment and orientation, (2) stabilization and rehabilitation, (3) reentry and employment, and (4) aftercare/transition. Each participant appears before the drug court judge biweekly throughout all four phases.

Phase I, assessment and orientation, lasts a minimum of 4 weeks. Residents go through an orientation and are provided any additional assessments they may need. Participants re restricted to the facility during this phase and receive random drug tests.

Phase II, stabilization and rehabilitation, lasts at least 12 weeks. During this period participants work on the treatment plans developed in Phase One. They also complete at least 200 hours of community service and begin a controlled process of community re-entry by attending five outside 12-Step group meetings per week. They also receive at least two random drug screens per month.

The third phase is re-entry and employment, and lasts at least 12 weeks. Participants work with their counselors to develop an aftercare plan, to find employment, and to further educational and vocational pursuits. A portion of each participant's salary to retained by the program to help offset expenses. AS s with Phase II, participants receive no less than 2 random drug screens monthly.

The final phase, aftercare/transition, lasts a minimum of six months. Paticipants, at this point considered graduates, move to transitional housing, returning to DC4 weekly for therapy and drug testing.

Rationale for Adding a Residential Component to Juvenile Drug Court

The advantages of adding a residential component to juvenile drug courts seem clear. First, given the experience of DC4, it seems likely that completion rates might be enhanced. Dealing with what is arguably a more difficult adult population, the residential program reports a retention rate of 65%. If juvenile treatment teams were able to identify likely candidates for residential treatment and make an appropriate recommendation to the court as does the DC4 adult team, more juveniles might complete the programs successfully. The residential component would need to be operated in a manner similar to that of DC4, be dedicated solely to drug court clients, and operated either by or in close partnership with the court.

Residential treatment would also provide alternative housing for juveniles who have no family or who are from toxic home environments. The Upper Cumberland Juvenile Drug Court study reported that 23.8% of treatment non-completers were placed in state custody. Many of these youth were placed in state custody because of delinquency charges brought during the course of their treatment. These were clearly non-compliant and would not have been eligible to move into a residential component. Others, however, were removed from their homes because those homes were abusive or neglectful. When the state welfare agency moved them to a foster home distance or other barriers prevented them from continuing. Had a residential component been present, juveniles doing well in the program might have been able to continue by moving from their homes and into the facility.

Finally, the addition of a residential component to juvenile drug courts would allow closer supervision and treatment for those for whom such is indicated. A phased process such as the one utilized by DC4 would allow closer interaction between juveniles and program staff, facilitating ongoing assessment and rapid intervention as the need arises.

Structure and Strategies for Adding Residential Components

Residential components might be added to existing juvenile drug courts in a variety of ways. Perhaps the most obvious method would be for the court to operate it as does DC4. Where this is not desirable or practical, local treatment providers might operate the facility, collaborating closely with the court as do other members of the treatment teams. Funding is a constant challenge for DC4, but it might prove easier to find for juvenile participants. State or federal funds from juvenile justice, child welfare, and substance abuse might be accessed both to cover startup costs and to provide operational funding after the facility has become operational. For example, Office of Juvenile Justice and Delinquency funds might become available to pay startup costs. Similarly, state juvenile justice and child welfare agencies could contract with the residential facility to pay for the youth in their custody.

CONCLUSION

Drug courts have been supported in the outcome literature as effective in reducing recidivism and use of substances for a variety of populations. The current study offers additional support, in this case for its effectiveness with juveniles. Despite the programs' successes, improvements may be possible. An example of one such possible improvement can be seen in the residential program of the Davidson County Drug Court. It is recommended that leaders in the field of adolescent residential treatment become involved in drug courts in their areas, and consider developing such residential programs in collaboration with them. Such endeavors seem likely to enhance the success of juvenile programs and seem practical from an operational and fiscal perspective.

REFERENCES

Belenko, S. (1998). Research on drug courts: A critical review. *National Drug Court Institute Review, 1.*

Cooper, C. (May, 2001). Juvenile drug court programs. NCJ 184744. (Available online: http://www.nchrs.gov/html/ojjdp/jaibg_2001_5_1/contents.html).

Finnigan, M. (1996). Societal Outcomes and Cost Savings of Drug and Alcohol Treatment in the State of Oregon. Salem, OR: Office of Alcohol and Drug Programs, Oregon Department of Human Resources.

Henggeler, S.W. (1999). Multisystemic Therapy: An overview of clinical procedures, outcomes, and policy implications. *Child Psychology and Psychiatry, 4*(1), 2-10.

Huddleston, C.W., Freeman-Wilson, K., Marlowe, D.B., & Roussel, A. (2005). *Painting the current picture: A national report card on drug courts and other problem-solving court programs in the United States.* Washington, DC: Bureau of Justice Assistance.

Jessor, R., & Jessor, S.L. (1977). *Problem behavior and psychosocial development: A longitudinal study of youth.* New York: Academic Press.

McPhail, M.W., & McNulty Weist, B. (1995). Combining alcohol and other drug abuse treatment with diversion for juveniles in the justice system. Treatment Improvement Protocol (TIP), Series 21. DHHS Publication No. (SMA) 95-3051. Washington, DC: Center for Substance Abuse Treatment.

Office of Applied Science. (2007). Number of Discharges from Substance Abuse Treatment age 12 or older and Percent who completed treatment course, United States, 2002-2004. Rockville, MD: Substance Abuse and Mental Health Services Administration.

RAND Corporation. (1997). Unpublished data. Santa Monica, CA; RAND Corporation.

Rempel, M., Fox-Kralstein, D., Cissner, A., Cohen, R., Labriola, M., Farole, D., Bader, A., & Magnani, M. (2003). *The New York State adult drug court evaluation: Policies, participants, and impacts.* New York, NY: Center for Court Innovation.

Roberts, M., Brophy, J., & Cooper, C. (March, 1997). The juvenile drug court movement. Office of Juvenile Justice and Delinquency Prevention Fact Sheet #59. Washington, DC: Office of Juvenile Justice and Delinquency Prevention.

Terry, III, W.C. (1998). Broward County's dedicated drug treatment court: From postadjudication to diversion. In Terry III, W.C. (ed.). *Judicial Change and Drug Treatment Courts: Case Studies in Innovation.* Beverly Hills, CA: Sage.

Cultural Considerations for Residential Treatment of Children and/or Adolescents

Lori K. Holleran Steiker, PhD

INTRODUCTION

Clinical settings have greatly increased their cognizance of cultural aspects of clients over the past few decades. Although ecological approaches to residential treatment have been prescribed and verbally embraced since the 1970s (Whitaker, 1979), the issue of culture has been scantly addressed in the research on youth residential treatment. Specific aspects of culture have been addressed such as organizational culture (Sawyer & Woodlock, 1995), trauma-sensitive culture (Farragher & Yanosy, 2005), and ethnicity as a variable of culture (Brady, 1995). However, little research has explored salient aspects of youth culture in residential treatment settings and therefore, too few evidence- based recommendations have been made. This may be due to the variety and diversity of such venues. It also may be due to the fact that most youth interventions are designed without consideration of and attention to cultural factors. In fact, many interventions are created by and for European Americans and tested primarily on this ethnic group. It has been suggested that the failure of many prevention and intervention programs can be traced to their lack of cultural sensitivity (Hansen, Miller, & Leukefeld, 1995; Palinkas et al., 1996).

Research indicates that tailoring an intervention to a target population can increase its effectiveness (Marsiglia et al., 2001). As a result, there has been a shift to ethnically-sensitive programs, based on the argument that cultural sensitivity enhances efforts and that ethnic matching maximizes program impact (Botvin et al., 1995). However, "culture," "acculturation," and "ethnicity" have been defined in various ways (Gutmann, 1999), and many studies approach ethnicity in a "glossed" fashion, denying the heterogeneity within groups and other contextual factors (Collins, 1995; Trimble, 1995). In fact, culture is a very complex phenomenon. Although observable similarities often exist among groups of people identified as of a common culture, significant differences are also common. A failure to acknowledge the differences can be just harmful as a failure to acknowledge the similarities. It is, therefore, imperative that practitioners become devoted students of culture, and of the individuals that compose cultures.

While some discussions of this subject aim at the goal of programs as "culturally appropriate," "culturally relevant," or "culturally competent," others note that culture is emergent, dynamic, and even curative in and of itself (Brady, 1995). In fact, both perspectives are accurate. It is important that practitioners and programs are able to interact effectively with members of other groups by being aware of and sensitive to their characteristics. It is equally vital, however, that they are aware of diversity and ongoing change and adaptation among members of specific cultures and their members. Experts have identified one of the likely causes of disparities in mental health service utilization is "cultural incongruity" (Cheung & Snowden, 1990), the opposite of cultural congruence which implies a fit between practice and culture. When the program does not fit the client in ways that are culturally important, the client may choose to avoid treatment ot may be unable to complete the program successfully. Rather than to try to achieve some magical point of cultural competence, it is more beneficial to agencies and clients to be culturally responsive (i.e., attending to not only culture, but the shifts and changes that occur in cultures constantly). This author maintains that the goal should be the "cultural grounding" of a program in the actual experiences of those that will receive the service (Holleran, Dustman, Reeves, & Marsiglia, 2002). In this scenario the practitioner is not only aware of cultural factors, but responsive to differences and change within groups both collectively and individually.

CULTURE IN AND OF A SETTING

Agencies, schools, and other organizations have two layers of culture–the culture within the setting (i.e., the demographic make-up of the population) and the culture of the setting (i.e., values, rules, and norms influenced by the philosophy and structure of the setting itself). These are in addition to, but interact with, smaller group cultures influenced by factors such as age, gender, ethnicity, custody status, and other factors.

Consistent with this realization, this author's research has prompted a much broader definition of culture than typically utilized. Instead of using ethnicity or socioeconomic status as a proxy for culture, it is recommended that researchers and clinicians consider the specific, unique, and ever-changing peer and organizational culture of unique settings. There is great diversity in the life experience of specific youth cultures such as homeless youth, incarcerated youth, GLBTQ youth, youth in alternative school settings (both disciplinary and by choice), and youth in unique cultural regions such as border cities, rural areas, etc. For example, research shows that rates of alcohol and other drug use are extremely high among homeless and street youth (Greene, Ennett, & Ringwalt, 1997; Kipke, Montgomery, Simon, & Iverson, 1997; Koopman, Rosario, & Rotheran-Borus, 1994), delinquent youth (Barnes, Welte, & Hoffman, 2002), youth from low SES environments (Eisner, 2002; Epstein, Botvin, & Diaz, 1995; Stewart, 2002), violent youth (Elickson, Saner & McGuigan, 1997), and adolescent mothers (Scafidi, Field, & Prodromidis, 1997). A history of drug use in combination with any of these other factors is likely to produce significant differences among those who might normally be considered part of the same group. For example, Latino youth who have been homeless and pregnant are likely to have adopted some characteristics of persons from those groups that distinguish them from Latino teens who have not had those experiences.

During drug prevention adaptation research and associated focus groups with adolescents in the unique settings listed above (Holleran Steiker & Hopson, 2007), youth noted unique cultural variations on the following aspects of their existence: substances of choice and availability, language for substances and use-related behaviors, social interactions, family interactions, preferred music, styles of interactions, and resistance strategies. For example, after two years of research in ten various youth settings, a group of incarcerated youth noted a common substance of abuse (e.g., "wet," or "dip" which was clarified to be cigarettes dipped in embalming fluid) that was not even mentioned by any other group in the study, despite the fact that nine out of ten of the agencies were in the same city. All these phenomena are arguably characteristics of a culture that is quite different from that of their peers.

CULTURE AND FAMILIES

Culture is also integrally tied with family. Exploring culture from a micro, meso and macro perspective points towards consideration of family attachments, boundaries, communication patters, as well as resources (e.g., community, extended family, financial, etc). There are few studies that examine the relationship between families and residential treatment programs (Baker, Heller, Blacher, & Pfeiffer, 1995; Johnson, 1999; Laufer, 1990; Shennum & Carlo, 1995) . In fact, a recent review of the literature produced only a single study, that of the relationship between families of color and residential treatment (Friesen, Kruzich, Longley, & Williams-Murphy, 2002). This paucity of literature underscores the danger of making uninformed about culture treatment. Clearly, it would be erroneous, and possibly undermining to treatment, to make assumptions about a family system by simply noting ethnic variables or SES. Yet, it would be equally harmful to ignore characteristics know to occur frequently within a culture. A culturally-grounded approach would be aware of those kinds of characteristics, and would assess families and clients for their presence. Yet a culturally-grounded approach would also be aware that individual and family experiences vary, and often produce diversity within groups or within families. In each case, these factors should certainly be explored in any assessment, as should family communication styles, behaviors, and beliefs.

CULTURE, DIVERSITY, AND INDIVIDUAL EXPERIENCE

Silva (1983) identified five life dimensions that interact within individual experiences to produce diversity. These dimensions include: (1) inherited endowment, (2) learned values and culture, (3) developmental histories, (4) specified patterns of problems, and (5) personalized styles of coping. Variation among and between these dimensions produces diversity between cultures, within families, and between individuals within cultures and families.

Understanding the sources of diversity can help practitioners anticipate differences among the groups in residential facilities. For example, the patterns of problems experienced by two Latino youths may be very different. One may be from a middle or upper class family of American citizens who immigrated to this country two generations ago. A second may be the child of a single, refugee parent who entered this country penniless and struggled with oppressive conditions in lower socioeconomic status neighborhood. Although these juveniles might have distinct similarities due to a common cultural background, their ways if interacting, looking at life, and reacting to challenges are likely to be very different. Understanding the background of each could help practitioners anticipate some of the strengths and deficits each will face during the treatment process and upon reentry into the community. These differences are also likely to affect choices made within an intervention (Atkinson, Morten, & Wing Sue, 1998; Ellis, Klepper, and Sowers, 2000).

RESIDENTIAL PEER CULTURE

For several decades, one of the major concerns with residential treatment for youth has been the potential for iatrogenic effects related to having troubled youth interacting together in a culture (Schaefer, 1980). There is currently a lot of interest in "peer contagion" (Gorman, 2007). Extended exposure to socially deviant peers is clearly a risk factor for some youth (Dodge, Dishion, & Lansford, 2006). Further, culture within a residential setting has been linked to specific behavioral issues among residents. For example, self mutilation has been well documented among incarcerated youth, gang members, and those in residential treatment (Derouin & Bravender, 2004).

At least two programs have been developed to try to offset the potential for the development of an antisocial culture among youth in treatment. These programs are Positive Peer Culture (PPC) and Positive Group Interaction (PGI).

Positive Peer Culture

Positive Peer Culture is an approach that has been utilized in residential treatment settings since the 1970s (Vorath & Brendtro, 1985; Davis, Hoffman, & Quigley, 1988; Donlevy & Weissman, 1992). PPC has holistic methods to work with youth in therapeutic settings (Springer, 2006). Brendtro and Ness (1991) described PPC as residential treatment that empowers youth as partners with staff in the problem solving process. Vorrath and Brendtro (1985) emphasize teaching youth to assume responsibility for mutual aid as well as responsibility for personal choices. Blaming and using excuses is not accepted as a mode of coping. With PPC, the peer group is viewed as a resource rather than a negative influence (Moody & Lupton-Smith, 2002). Residents are encouraged both to behave prosocially and to support others in prosocial behavior. By helping others, a group member's sense of self worth increases (Vorrath & Brendtro, 1985). Small discussion groups are used to increase respect, trust, and openness among residents. The intention of a PPC is to "replace a negative culture with a more positive one" (Moody & Lupton-Smith, 2002).

Early research into PPC's effectiveness reported increases in self-awareness, positive self-image, increased ability to identify personal problems and make more rational decisions, and a higher level of concern for oneself and others (Tannehill, 1987). Early research on PPC programs also demonstrated positive and lasting changes in the self esteem, locus of control, moral values, and academic achievement of members as a result of in-group interventions (Brendtro & Wasmund, 1988; Davis et al., 1988). Vorath and Brendtro (1985) called PPC, "a total system for building positive youth subcultures." More recent research findings show that this intervention in residential settings is successful when the variable "openness to social relationships" is present among the youth. It also revealed that, when residents lack the capacity for relatedness, PPC is less likely to be successful (Lee, 1996).

POSITIVE GROUP INTERACTION

More recently, a variation entitled Positive Group Interaction (PGI) has been developed. PGI is a peer-based method of infusing residential treatment with the nuances of the peer group being treated. According to Vollmer (2005), the focus on peer culture allows for "the creation of a safe and healthy environment, the establishment of an atmosphere of trust, and the use of a residential treatment group as a powerful force in order to achieve behavior modification of its individual group members."

Programs such as PGI should be adopted in residential facilities, but must incorporate awareness of and sensitivity to the culture of and cultures within the group. Further, the culture of the facility must be such that practitioners are rewarded for promoting the program and related culturally responsive or culturally grounded activities.

RECOMMENDATIONS FOR RESIDENTIAL TREATMENT SETTINGS

As noted above, agencies, schools, and other organizations are commonly conceptualized as having two layers of culture: the culture within the setting (i.e., the demographic make-up of the population) and the culture of the setting itself (i.e., values, rules, and norms influenced by the philosophy and structure of the setting itself). Culture is present and active in residential facilities in other ways as well. For instance, there is likely to be a culture among the residents, a culture among the employees, and a culture that exists between residents and employees. Further, the ethnic and family cultures of residents affect interactions and perceptions among residents and between residents and employees.

In order to engage, impact, and intervene on youth in residential settings, it is important to carefully examine the intersection of all these cultures and aspects of culture. Institutions should consciously assess both their organizational culture and the culture that exists among their residents. They should be alert to changes that occur within those cultures. For example, changes within the organizational culture may occur after the retirement of a key employee. Changes within the resident culture may occur when several juveniles graduate simultaneously or in response to an influx of new residents.

There are instruments that have been established and validated which can help to assess the culture of an agency. For example, the School Success Profile Learning Organization or SSP-LO (Bowen et al., 2006) has been easily adapted to cultures other than schools and it assesses such areas as staff's team orientation, innovation, involvement, information flow, tolerance for error, results orientation, common purpose, respect, cohesion, trust, mutual support, and optimism (Bowen et al., 2006). The outcomes of the measure can be used to determine the styles and attitudes of the milieu. A range of instruments with differing characteristics are available to those who are interested in organizational culture, all of which have varied strengths and utilities (Scott, Mannion, Davies, & Marshall, 2003).

Strength-based rather than pathology-based interventions are critical with youth who face behavioral and psychological challenges (Laursen, 2000). Familiarity with the cultural backgrounds of individual youth can allow treatment personnel to help those juveniles draw upon the strengths inherent in their culture. Similarly, it can provide opportunities to link youth with external cultural resources that may provide hope, self-esteem, and encouragement.

Becoming aware of and responsive to the various cultures in their environment allows practitioners to better meet the needs of all individuals and groups. In the field of education the term "culturally responsive" is often used to describe this condition. Social services tend to utilize the term culturally competent, implying that that one might at some point be perfectly versed in a culture. Whatever term is chosen, being responsive or competent requires awareness of the complex and dynamic nature of culture, of the ways in which it changes, waxes and wanes of trends, and how it is affected by the inevitable discovery of powerful, new information. These dynamics require that constant and consistent effort be made by program staff to be aware of and responsive to changes in the culture within their facility and variations within the culture of the children and adolescents that serve.

In order to implement a Positive Peer Culture model, clinicians should embrace a strengths-based perspective. According to Moody and Lupton-Smith (2000), practical recommendations for implementation include the following: small group size (i.e., one adult leader, with nine youth (12-18 year-olds), and of the same-sex (Vorrath & Brendtro, 1985); meetings held three to five times weekly for approximately one to one and a half hours (Tannehill, 1987); trained adult leaders acting as limit setters, listeners, and coaches in responsibility for self; and family members are not be in the same group (Vorrath & Brendtro, 1985). When assignments are given to group, emphasis is placed upon group rather than individual reward (Laufenberg, 1987). The experts not that it is important that clinicians, when considering Positive Peer Culture interventions, evaluate (1) whether the clients have the necessary basic social skills, and (2) whether resources are available (Moody & Lupton-Smith,

1999). These are necessary ingredients for successful implementation of this model.

CONCLUSION

For decades, it has been known that the most important component in interventions with youth is an honest, genuine and warm connection with those that are receiving services (Yalom & Rand, 1966; Miller & Rollnick, 1991). However, culture is often overlooked or underestimated as an ingredient in therapeutic relationships. Often, it is oversimplified, undervalued, assumed. In order to truly attend to the culture of youth, it is critical that clinicians and researchers utilize the youth themselves as experts on their own life experiences (Gosin, Marsiglia, & Hecht, 2003; Holleran Steiker, 2006).

Properly understood and competently managed, culture can be a healing ingredient in a residential environment. Practitioners must be aware of its multiple layers and its inherent diversity in order to optimize its therapeutic benefit. They must understand the culture within the facility as well as the culture of the facility. They must understand and be sensitive to the cultural characteristics children and youth bring to treatment: those of their ethnicity, those of their family, and those they bring as individuals. Further, they must be sensitive to factors that may promote the development of unhealthy cultural components and find ways to minimize those effects. At least two useful, evidence-based programs exist that can provide a framework for culturally-grounded residential practice. These are Positive Peer Culture and Positive Group Interaction.

REFERENCES

Atkinson, Morten, & Wing Sue. (1998). *Counseling American Minorities*. New York: McGraw Hill Publishers.

Baker, B.L., Heller, T.L., Blacher, J., & Pfeiffer, S.I. (1995). Staff attitudes toward family involvement in residential treatment centers for children. *American Psychiatric Association, 46*, 60-65.

Barnes, G.M., Welte, J.W., & Hoffman, J.H. (2002). Relationship of alcohol use to delinquency and illicit drug use in adolescents: Gender, age, and racial/ethnic differences. *Journal of Drug Issues, 32*(1), 153-178.

Botvin, G.J., Baker, E., & Dusenbury, L. (1995). Long-term followup results of a randomized drug abuse prevention trial in a white middle class population. *Journal of the American Medical Association, 273* (14), 1106-1112.

Bowen, G.L., Rose, R.A., & Ware, W.B. (2006). The reliability and validity of the School Success Profile Learning Organization Measure. *Evaluation and Program Planning, 29*, 97-104.

Brady, M. (1995). Culture in treatment, culture as treatment. A critical appraisal of developments in addictions programs for indigenous North Americans and Australians. *Social Science & Medicine*, 41(11), 1487-98.

Brendtro, L.K. & Ness, A.E. (1991). Extreme interventions for extreme behavior: Peer-assisted behavior management in group treatment programs. *Journal Child and Youth Care Forum*, 20(3), 171-181.

Carlo, P. & Shennum, W.A. (1989). Family reunification efforts that work: A three year follow-up study of children in *residential treatment. Journal Child and Adolescent Social Work Journal*, 6(3), 211-216.

Cheung, F.K. & Snowden, L.R. (1990). Community mental health and ethnic minority populations. *Journal Community Mental Health Journal*, 26(3), 277-291.

Collins, R.L. (1995). Issues of ethnicity in research on prevention of substance abuse. In G.J. Botvin, S. Schinke, Orlandi, M.A. (1995). *Drug abuse prevention with multiethnic youth.* Sage: Thousand Oaks, London, New Dehli.

Davis, G.L., Hoffman, R.G., & Quigley, R. (1988). Self-concept change and positive peer culture in adjudicated delinquents. *Journal Child and Youth Care Forum*, 17(3), 137-145.

Dodge, K.A., Dishion, T.J., & Lansford, J.E. (2006). Deviant Peer Influences in Intervention and Public Policy for Youth. *Social Policy Report*, XX(1), 3-19.

Donlevy, J.G. & Weissman, G. (1992). Integrating Positive Peer Culture into the Residential Treatment Center and Public School Curriculum: Suggestions for Practice. *Journal of Correctional Education*, 43(4), 166-70.

Derouin, A. & Bravender, T. (2004). Living on the edge: the current phenomenon of self-mutilation in adolescents. *American Journal of Maternal Child Nursing*, 29(1), 12-18.

Eisner, M. (2002). Crime, problem drinking, and drug use: Patterns of problem behaviors in cross-national perspective. *The Annals of the American Academy of Political and Social Science, 580*, 201-225.

Elickson, P., Saner, H., & McGuigan, K.A. (1997). Profiles of violent youth: substance use and other concurrent problems. *American Journal of Public Health, 87,* 985-991.

Ellis, R.A., Klepper, T.D., & Sowers, K.M. (2000b). Building a foundation for effective intervention: Understanding Hispanic juveniles and their families. *Journal for Juvenile Justice and Detention Services*, 15(2), 26-39.

Epstein, J.A., Botvin, G. J., & Diaz, T. (1995). The role of social factors and individual characteristics in promoting alcohol use among inner-city minority youth. *Journal of Studies on Alcohol, 56*, 39-46.

Farragher, B. & Yanosy, S. (2005). Creating a trauma-sensitive culture in residential treatment. *Therapeutic Community*, 26(1), 97-113.

Friesen, B.J., Kruzich, J.M., Longley, M.J., & Williams-Murphy, T. (2002). Voices of African American Families: Perspectives on Residential Treatment. *Social Work*, 47(4), 461-70.

Gorman, D. (2007). Unpublished conversation with researcher, Feb. 19, 2007.

Gosin, M., Marsiglia, F.F., & Hecht, M. L. (2003). Keepin' it R.E.A.L.: A drug resistance curriculum tailored to the strengths and needs of pre-adolescents of the Southwest. *Journal of Drug Education*, 33(2), 119-142.

Greene, J.M., Ennett, S.T., & Ringwalt, C.L. (1997). Substance use among runaway and homeless youth in three sample. *American Journal of Public Health*, 87, 229-235.

Gutmann, M.C. (1999). Ethnicity, alcohol, and acculturation. *Social Science and Medicine*, 48, 173-184.

Hansen, W.B., Miller, T.W., & Leukefeld, C.G. (1995). Prevention research recommendations: Scientific integration for the 90's. *Drugs & Society*, 8(3/4), 161-167.

Holleran Steiker, L.K. (2006). Consulting with the experts: Utilizing adolescent input in substance use prevention efforts. *Social Perspectives/Perspectivas Sociales*, 8(1), 53-66.

Holleran Steiker, L.K. & Hopson, L.M. (2007). Evaluation of Culturally Adapted, Evidence-Based Substance Abuse Prevention Programs for Older Adolescents in Diverse Community Settings. Advancing Adolescent Health Conference. Presentation at The University of Texas at Austin, Center for Health Promotion Research. February 28.

Holleran, L.K., Dustman, P., Reeves, L., & Marsiglia, F.F. (2002). Creating culturally grounded videos for substance abuse prevention: A dual perspective on process. *Journal of Social Work Practice in the Addictions*, 2(1), 55-78.

Johnson, M.M. (1999). Multiple dimensions of family-centered practice in residential group care: Implications regarding the roles of stakeholders. *Journal Child and Youth Care Forum*, 28,(2), 123-141.

Kipke, M.D., Montgomery, S.B., Simon, R.R., & Iverson, E.F. (1997). Substance abuse disorders among runaway and homeless youth. *Substance Use and Misuse*, 32, 965-982.

Koopman, C., Rosario, M., & Rotheram-Borus, M.J. (1994). Alcohol and drug use and sexual behaviors placing runaways at risk for HIV infection. *Addictive Behaviors*, 19, 95-103.

Laufenberg, R. (1987). Positive peer culture: A peer group approach to behavior change. *Journal of Correctional Education*, 38(4),138-43.

Laufer, Z. (1990). Family ties as viewed by child care and treatment personnel in residential settings for children aged 6–14. *Journal Child and Youth Care Forum*, 19(1), 49-57.

Laursen, E.K. (2000). Strength-based practice with children. *Reclaiming Children and Youth*, 9(2), 70.

Lee, R.E. (1996). FIRO-B scores and success in a positive peer-culture residential treatment program *Psychological Reports*, 78(1), 215-20.

Marsiglia, F.F., Kulis, S., & Hecht, M.L. (2001). Ethnic labels and ethnic identity as predictors of drug use and drug exposure among middle school students in the Southwest. *Journal of Research on Adolescence*, 11(1), 21-48.

Miller, W.R. & Rollnick, S. (1991). *Motivational Interviewing: Preparing People to Change Addictive Behavior*. New York: Guilford Press.

Moody, E.E. & Lupton-Smith, H.S. (1999). Interventions with juvenile offenders: Strategies to prevent acting out behavior. *Journal of Addictions & Offender Counseling*, (20)1, 2-14.

Moody, E. & Lupton-Smith, H. (2002). Interventions with juvenile offenders: Strategies to prevent acting out behavior. *Journal of Addictions & Offender Counseling*, 20(1), 2-14.

Palinkas, L.A., Atkins, C.J., Jerreira, D., & Miller, C. (1996). Effectiveness of social skills training form primary and secondary prevention of drug use in high-risk female adolescents. *Preventive Medicine*, 25, 692-701.

Sawyer, D.A & Woodlock, D.J. (1995). An organizational culture paradigm for effective residential treatment. *Journal Administration and Policy in Mental Health and Mental Health Services Research*, 22(4), 437-446.

Scafidi, F.A., Field, T., & Prodromidis, M. (1997). Psychosocial stressors of drug-abusing disadvantaged adolescent mothers. *Adolescence*, 32, 93-100.

Schaefer, C. (1980). The impact of the peer culture in the residential treatment of youth. *Adolescence*, 15(60), 831-45.

Scott, T., Mannion, R., Davies, H., & Marshall, M. (2003). The quantitative measurement of organizational culture in health care: A review of the available instruments. *Health Services Research*, 38(3), 923-945.

Silva, J.S. (1983). Cross-cultural and cross-ethnic assessment. In C. Gibson (Ed.). *Our kingdom stands on brittle glass* (pp. 59-66). Silver Springs, MD: National Association of Social Workers.

Springer, D. (2006). Substance abuse treatment for juvenile delinquents: Promising and not-so-promising practices in the U.S. *Social Perspectives/Perspectivas Sociales*, 8(1), 23-52.

Stewart, C. (2002). Family factors of low-income African-American youth associated with substance use: an exploratory analysis. *Journal of Ethnicity in Substance Abuse*, 1(1), 97-111.

Tannehill, R.L. (1987). Employing a modified positive peer culture treatment approach in a state youth center. *Journal of Offender Counseling, Services and Rehabilitation*, 12, 113-129.

Trimble (1995). Toward an understanding of ethnicity and ethnic identity, and their relationship with drug use research. In G.J. Botvin, S. Schinke, & M.A. Orlandi (Eds.). *Drug Abuse Prevention with Multiethnic Youth* (pp. 28-45). Thousand Oaks, CA: Sage.

Vollmer, T. (2005). Creating a peer-directed environment: An approach to making residential treatment a unique experience by using the power of peer groups. *Journal Child and Youth Care Forum*, 34(3), 175-193.

Vorath, H.H. & Brendtro, L.K. (1985). *Positive peer culture*. New York: Aldrine de Gryter.

Wasmund, W.C. (1988). Peer group treatment for troubled youth: The social climates of peer group and other residential programs. *Journal Child and Youth Care Forum*, 17(3), 146-155.

White, W.L. (1996). *Pathways from the culture of addiction to the culture of recovery: a travel guide for addiction professionals* (2nd ed.), Hazelden: Center City, MN.

Whittaker, J.K. (1979). *Caring for Troubled Children: Residential Treatment in a Community Context.* New York: Aldine de Gruyter.

Yalom, I.D. & Rand, K. (1966). Compatibility and cohesiveness in therapy groups. *Archives of General Psychiatry,* 15(3), 267-75.

Manhood Seekers Camp:
A Proposal for a Culturally-Centered Camp Intervention

Gregory Washington, PhD
Roderick J. Watts, PhD
Jerry Watson, PhD

INTRODUCTION

Culturally centered camp programs can provide a unique intervention through which vulnerable African-American male youth in residential child welfare placements could make gains in their emotional and social functioning. The therapeutic value of creating activities that promote healthy identity development and build upon specific cultural strengths may be a valuable area that is missing from the literature related to camps as therapeutic interventions. This paper expands traditional camp opportunities by proposing a culturally-centered approach for interventions that emphasizes same gender, race and ethnicity characteristics. Training guidelines are suggested for camp facilitators to enhance cultural awareness and promote the incorporation of culturally specific activities. The experiences and impressions of camp facilitators who have piloted a culturally-centered camp for at-risk African-American are described and discussed.

There may not be a great appreciation in the literature on camps and recreation programs of the value of camps as venues for effective interventions (Breton, 1990; Gentry, 1984; Redl, 1966; Schwartz, 1960). There does appear to be growing literature that implores practitioners to return to camps as feasible and vital interventions for youth with learning disabilities and related psychosocial problems (Collins, 2003; Michalski & Mishna, 2003; Mishna, Michalski, & Cummings, 2001). The evaluation of such camp interventions resulted in some promising findings related to the enhancement of social competence, self- confidence, self-esteem and a decreased sense of social isolation (Michalski, Mishna, Worthington, & Cummings, 2003). However, there is a paucity of literature describing the race, culture and ethnicity influences on campers and the camp facilitators. The absence of this information is problematic for social workers in child welfare arenas with large ethnic minority populations because they frequently utilize summer camps as part of a cadre of special service experiences for children in foster home and group home placements. Child welfare professionals seek camp experiences to enrich the quality of out of home placements and research findings that identify African-Americans youth disproportionately experience these out of home placements (Logan, 2000). These are youth who have frequently have experienced emotional neglect and been exposed to violent behavior that may contribute to greater risk for poor school performance, psychosocial problems, violent and delinquent behavior (Fagan & Wilkinson, 1998; Singer, Anglin, Song, & Lunghofer, 1995; Schott Foundation, 2006). These youth may be in need of therapeutic services such as therapeutic camp programs. Evaluations of camp programs for children and adolescents with learning disabilities and psychosocial problems offer compelling illustrations of how camps can be effective contexts for social group work interventions but a review of the literature did not produce literature that addresses the context of race, ethnicity and culture. There is also ambiguity concerning the difference between these terms which are often used interchangeably.

The similarity-attraction paradigm (Byrne, 1971) and Ogbu's (1990) framework for mentoring minority youth may have relevancy for understanding the ethnic similarity dynamics between camp participants and camp facilitators. Byrne and Ogbu have presented explanations that suggest ethnic similarity is a factor to consider when structuring therapeutic camps that utilize the relationship dynamics between the camp participants and camp facilitators to promote therapeutic change.

The importance of same gender camp facilitator and camp participant matches as it relates to identity development is another area not adequately addressed in social work camp intervention literature. The impact of same gender and cross gender relationships may vary in their impact on youth. Identifying factors related to attitudes, motivations and behaviors of potential African-American men camp facilitators is important because African-American boys may benefit from therapeutic camp interventions facilitated by these men. The experiences and impressions of the camp facilitators is another area that has not been reported in the literature.

This paper seeks to fill those gaps in the literature. First theoretical perspectives on the roles of race, ethnicity and culture in therapeutic relationships are considered. Second, theories and research findings that discuss gender and ethnicity in therapeutic relationships are reviewed. Third, the impressions of African-African camp facilitators in a culturally-centered camp for African- American boys are examined and future directions for practitioners are discussed.

LITERATURE REVIEW: RACE, ETHNICITY AND CULTURE

Discussions regarding race, ethnicity and culture frequently proceed without the understanding of what the differences are between these terms. The significance of the most controversial of the three, race, has been debated as an outdated term with declining significance and simultaneously as a term with increasing significance in light of its history and usage as a social concept to oppress and justify special privilege to groups of people (Green, 1982; Healey, 1995; Logan, Freeman, & McRoy, 1990; Willie, 1978; Wilson, 1978). The clear biological and genetic heritage characteristics once thought to exist between racial groups have been proven by physical anthropologists to be not very clear or distinct at all while at the same time the social reality of different experiences between people identified as white and any other color has been consistently verified (Healey, 1995). This debate prompted the use of the term ethnic groups to describe the differences between people.

Ethnicity has been defined as groups of individuals who share a common culture, nationality, history or religion (Robinson & Howard-Hamilton, 2000). Culture can be a difficult concept to grasp because is encompasses all of what we regularly do. It refers to the characteristic life-ways of a people: the way they think, feel and behave (Chestang, 1976). Culture also includes the traditional values and ideas learned, shared and transmitted from generation to generation and helps interpret existence and organizes life (Gordon, 1964; Linton, 1945; Kroeber & Kluckholm, 1952). The potential negative consequences for youth that are subjected to the cultural suppression of African and African-American history are being recognized. There is a rich history of African societies and African-American accomplishments influenced by men of African descent that could be inaccessible to the young African-American male if cultural suppression takes place. It is suggested that almost all knowledge about Africa received by African-American male youth has been filtered by Europeans and consequently is Eurocentric (Asante, 1998). In other words, it has been modified by Europeans or

European Americans for the purpose of fitting the African into the European world. Over 100 years ago, Dubois (1903) identified the negation and subjugation of African-American culture as a continual process in the United States that has required first African slaves and later the African Americans to negate their cultural essence. Socialization that is influenced by cultural suppression could be a factor that leads to emotional conflict and stress for African-Americans, particularly at risk young males (Akbar, 1981; Stevenson, 1994).

Increasingly social scientists have chosen to distinguish between human groups on the basis of cultural differences versus race or ethnicity and are increasingly more conscious of the role that cultural values play in influencing the psychological processes and behavioral outcomes of diverse populations. Many researchers who look at health disparities such as violence that impacts young African-American males utilize a broad definition that includes a common heritage or set of beliefs and norms and the acknowledge that culture is dynamic in nature (US Department of Health and Human Services, 2001).

GENDER, ETHNICITY AND IDENTITY DEVELOPMENT

The gender-intensification hypothesis (Hill & Lynch, 1983) articulates the argument that gender specific beliefs and behaviors increase during adolescence. According to Erickson (1968) per his stages of psychosocial development, gender role characteristics become more salient around puberty and present the child with the challenge of industry-versus-inferiority. At this pre-adolescent stage, the need is not just for behavioral competence, but more importantly, a sense of mastery. In adolescence, the developmental challenge becomes identity-versus-role-confusion as through adolescence the child progresses toward manhood and contends with the question, "Who am I?" African-American boys in socially and economically poor communities may experience this development differently and be at risk of experiencing problems in healthy identity development due in part to societal stigma related to the black male image and the characteristics of their economically disadvantaged environments (Hutchinson, 1994; Spencer, 1990). Assisting in the successful resolution of these challenges at the early stages of human development is the most optimal point of intervention because it is harder to meet the challenges of the later stages unless the earlier ones have been resolved successfully (Erickson, 1968).

Complicating the challenge of healthy black male identity development for the youth in America's poor inner-city communities is the exodus of upper class and middle-class families, the presence of drug related crime, and the incarceration of men and the resulting lack of available healthy African-American male role models. This has contributed to a polarization that leaves many lower-class families with schools and social institutions with fewer resources.

Healthy psychological development of African Americans has included the challenges of addressing the forces that have either attempted to erase their cultural consciousness or contributed to Nigrescence, a maladaptive or unhealthy African-American identity (Akbar, 1981; Cross, Parham, & Helms, 1985). Traditional models of identity development largely ignore cultural patterns of coping and other unique experiences and characteristics of people of color. It is hypothesized that a multifaceted theoretical formulation is required to understand the identity development of children of color (Spencer & Markstrom-Adams, 1990). The Nigrescence models of Cross, Parham, and Helms (1985) describe the development of black identity and are among the few culturally centered models that have provided the foundation for research that has attempted to describe the identity development of African-American youth. It was long ago suggested by the great African-American educator and historian Carter G. Woodson (1933) that for African-American boys, role models may be especially important. He somewhat prophetically envisioned a hostile environment for young African-American males resulting from a colonized educational system void of any examples of positive, strong African-American males. The current rates of suspensions, special education and incarceration may be evidence of the hostile environment Woodson envisioned.

Many African-centered scholars suggest the degree to which young African-American males identify with and embrace their African and African-American heritage relates to their degree of social health and vulnerability to social problems (Asante, 1980; Akbar, 1981; Karenga, 1988; Nobles, 1984; Oliver, 1989; Schiele, 2000). If this is true, African-American men could be a valuable resource in efforts to engage

African-American boys in group interventions that promote value clarification and healthy identity development. Research related to group interventions that emphasize African and African-American culture is sparse but includes promising findings (Washington et al., 2007; Utsey, Howard, & Williams, 2003).

A THERAPEUTIC CULTURALLY CENTERED CAMP

In 2003 Anasi, Inc., and four African-American men in their 40s, were commissioned by a private child welfare agency in Atlanta to develop and operate a four day camp for African-American boys at various stages of transition to permanent homes. There were also two young African-American men in their 20s trained and commissioned as camp facilitators for what was intended to be a camp that would emphasize assets and characteristics required to be healthy African-American young men. The fourteen boys who were camp participants were all residing in temporary out of home residential settings for youth who had special medical and psychological needs. A training model was designed by Anasi to prepare the men and identify an activities agenda that would emphasize positive aspects of African and African-American culture. The agenda was informed through the human development theories and research findings identified earlier that promote identity development and socialization by mentors who were of similar ethnic background. An ethnic similarity therapeutic approach is also collaborated by theory and research findings supporting the hypothesis that clinical benefit is greater among ethnic minority clients paired with an ethically similar versus dissimilar therapists (Halliday-Boykins, Schoenwald, & Letourneau, 2005; Sue, Fujino, Hu, Takeuchi, & Zane, 1991).

Training Model

The six African-American men identified as camp facilitators received six hours of training prior to the beginning of the camp that included orientation to Afrocentric concepts. Consistent with an Afrocentric worldview, this training emphasized collectivity and the spiritual nature of the relationship between camp facilitators and the boys. Training included opportunities to do self-exploration and clarify protocol for interacting with the mentees and processing the interactions. The basics of human development tasks in the preadolescent and adolescent years were identified in training and were referenced during daily camp facilitator processing sessions.

The training emphasized opportunities to discuss and explore male role models in the African-American community. It is suggested that the void of such models could be a negative factor in the educational success, behavior problems and the potential for some African-Americans to have a more "externalized loci of control" (Rodney & Mupier, 1999; Rodney, Tachia, & Rodney, 1999; Wilson, 1987). The men were encouraged to share personal strategies for navigating stereotypical views and community influences that tend to demonize African-American males.

The social workers, clinicians and students selected as camp facilitators were engaged in exercises to specifically address black male negative valuation issues because it is important to address the potentially racist socialization experiences of men who work with African-American boys (Caldwell & White, 2001). Dyadic and experiential exercises allowed for the sharing of personal life experiences that included the successful resolution of fatherhood, racism, oppression, gang involvement, addictions and other health issues. While disclosure of some of these experiences to the boys was not appropriate and did not occur, the men discussed challenging life experiences among themselves and how these experiences could contribute to the developing healthy relationships with the boys. The youngest men provided insider knowledge about gangs, and youth and hip-hop culture that was a valuable tool for informing the older men and building "street credibility" or rapport with the boys who tended to be very aware of urban inner city youth culture.

Anasi Camp Agenda

The goal of the camp was to engage the boys in activities designed to clarify characteristics and values related to healthy African-American males. The camp agenda was influenced by the ground-breaking work of Nathan and Julia Hare (1985). A central strategy of the group intervention was infusing the themes of the *Nguzo Saba*, which is Swahili for "Seven Principles," into the discussion and interactions between men and boys. The Nguzo Saba includes principles grounded in African-centered, Pan-Africanist and socialist thought (Karenga, 1988). Dr. Maulana Karenga conceptualized these principles as a vehicle for African-Americans to affirm their African ancestry and promote positive cultural traditions and lessons from that ancestry (Azibo, 1996; Karenga, 1988). The *Nguzo Saba* is incorporated into the application of NTU psychotherapy as a means to help clients have a guideline for healthy living (Phillips, 1996). From the Afrocentric perspective it is the concentration on themes, such as unity, spirituality and collectivity that are crucial to healthy identity development in African-American male youth. The *Nguzo Saba* (Seven Principles) follows:

UMOJA (Unity)
KUJICIHAGULIA (Self-Determination)
UJIMA (Collective Work and Responsibility)
UJAMAA (Co-Operative Economics)
NIA (Purpose)
KUUMBA (Creativity)
IMANI (Faith) (Azibo, 1996: 83).

The daily activities began at 8:30 am with the camp facilitators' preparation of breakfast for the boys. There was also individual interaction with boys who needed help with medication and dressing appropriately. The agenda and principles emphasized the following:

8:30am-10:00am
Principle: *Imani/Faith*

Relaxation Exercises/Eye Opener meditation
Discussion topic:
Wellness/Safety/Spirituality
Personal Wellness Begins in the
Past/current health status
   Safety, Nutrition and Lifestyle
   Exercise: Deep breathing and music

11:15am-12:30pm
Principle: *Kuumba/Creativity*

Therapeutic recreation activity
Hiking,
Rafting, or
Fishing

12:45pm-1:15pm
Principles: Nguza Saba

Discussion topic: Community Life and African Values

Exploring Values (WWIII exercise or cartoon)

Personal Values

Traditional Values (Comic books)

1:30pm-3:00pm
Principle: Kuumba/Creativity

Therapeutic recreation activity
Biking,

Horseback riding, or

Hiking

4:10pm-5:00pm
Principles: Ujima/Collective responsibility and Umoja/Unity)

Preparation for Community Campfire
Getting In Touch "Inner" Selves

Spirituality and nature

Community service project

Community wellness

5:00pm Community Campfire
Principle: Nia/Purpose
Breathing and relaxation

Stress management
Lessons learned today

Data Collection and Findings

An outside evaluator was present to observe key activities and dialogue with the camp facilitators and capture their impressions and reactions process the rating sheets. The small sample size of men precluded a rigorous quantitative outcome evaluation, but it was possible to focus on process evaluation. The aim of the process evaluation follows with evaluation findings, limitations, recommendations and implications. Prior to departure for the campsite, facilitators used forms developed by the evaluator to specify program goals and activities. During and after the camp they provided written documentation on rating sheets about the activities along with their reactions and judgments (Table 1).

TABLE 1. Goal Areas
#1
Educational and Vocational Options
#2
Personal Strengths and Clarity on Nguzo Saba Values
#3
Critical Thinking on Race and Manhood
#4
Constructive Group Participation and Pro-social Behavior

The aim of a process evaluation was to analyze and document the program implementation process by identifying key program activities and operational aspects of the program. The findings relate to the impressions of the camp facilitators particularly as they attempted to clarify characteristics and values for positive African-American men. The men had three options for rating the camp activities on the rating sheets (raters coded 1, 2 or 3 respectively for each camp activity).

1. *We made little progress toward this goal, and this activity did not contribute much.*
2. *We made good progress toward this goal and this activity was valuable.*
3. *We made more progress toward the goal than I expected, and this activity made a very important contribution.*

Many of the camp activities were outdoor recreational activities intended to challenge the young men in novel ways and to build relationships with the staff and among the participants (rafting, biking, etc.). Several other activities included an emphasis on African culture, especially those cultural concepts that encouraged pro-social behavior (collective work and responsibility, for example). Reflection on their experience was encouraged in daily evening discussions and through journaling.

Staff rated the value of nearly every camp activity very highly. Only once did an activity get rated "1" (i.e., the lowest rating on the 3 point scale). This was the comic book reading activity related to the discussion about values. Most others were rated 3: *"We made more progress toward the goal than I expected, and this activity made a very important contribution."*

The following are the evaluator's direct observations which began on day three and ended on day four. The group was on the move most of the day, going to the scheduled activities and managing the logistics of transportation and meals. The horseback riding was challenging (but within the limits) of the youngsters who participated, and those who did not feel up to the challenge were allowed to sit out the activity. The camp facilitators had the skills and patience to keep things running smoothly and to use conflict or problem behavior of the young men as opportunities to reinforce the camp's psychosocial and cultural themes.

The theme heard most often was Umoja (unity) and reminders that the group was to work collectively as a community. The evaluator and the facilitators felt the wide age ranges of the boys, 8-14, sometimes negatively impacted their ability to consistently communicate complex concepts.

The highlight of each evening at the camp was a ritual meeting with a "council of elders" complete with drumming and campfire. On night three all the men brought the boys before them, one by one and out of earshot of the others, to quiz them on what they had learned during their stay about themselves and about some of the cultural ideas discussed. The camp facilitators prepared for the encounters by discussing each participant before he arrived, and what they decided what to ask and what feedback to give the boys about their actions. The camp facilitators were impressed by the power of the nightly campfires. They observed that while recall and insight of the boys was uneven at times, but they always seemed in awe of the event and they were consistently serious and respectful of the proceedings.

A few additional observations: a number of camp facilitators said in informal discussions that the time and energy spent in food preparation was distracting from their work with the young people. Indeed, it was evident that the logistics of transporting all the food they would need and then preparing it and cleaning up was a major operation. The boys were not involved in this responsibility, so it rotated among camp facilitators.

Curiously, although staff identified the youngsters' family relationships as important, the concluding family "feast" on day four was not evaluated. The evaluator did not stay for the feast with the young men's families and there were no camp facilitator comments about it, so it is unclear how this seemingly major event fit with program goals.

LIMITATIONS AND IMPLICATIONS FOR FUTURE PRACTICE AND RESEARCH

The major limitations of this study are due to the small very heterogeneous sample and missing data on youth behavior. Consequently, inferences that the observed improvements in the boys were due to the camp experience are highly speculative. Despite the significant limitations in this pilot effort at creating camp experiences for a newly formed group of young African American men, the results are encouraging. Future culturally-centered camp interventions efforts should evaluate the influence on youth participants. The following are also suggestions that have implications for future practice and research:

1. Use the camp experience as a team and relationship building event at the beginning of the group's formation, or as a culminating rite of passage event to mark an achievement in the group's development. Using it as an isolated event for a group that has no significant history or future, and probably weakens its potential impact.
2. Work collaboratively with caregivers and camp facilitators from the start. Try to build a consensus on priority program areas and have the priority themes reinforced consistently in the training sessions with the young men before and after the camp.
3. Reduce the variation in age of camp participants. Although there are some suggestions that younger as well as older youngsters can benefit from this experience, there seems to be clearer benefits for the older boys. A more homogenous age cohort was suggested to allow more dialogue among the boys. This is also consistent with the age cohort structure of traditional African rites of passage. Nonetheless, a separate group for younger boys is also worth considering.
4. Maintain as high a staff to participant ratio as possible. This seemed to be an important advantage in managing the youngsters. Highly trained staff may not be necessary; the use of properly prepared undergraduate college camp facilitators should be considered. These mentors could develop relationships with the young men before and after the camp that would provide psychosocial support, and they could also reinforce the ideas covered in the camp.

REFERENCES

Akbar, N. (1981). Mental disorder among African-Americans. *Black Books Bulletin*, 7(2), 18-25.

Asante, M.K. (1980). *Afrocentricity: The theory of social change*. Buffalo, NY: Amulefi Publishing Company.

Asante, M.K. (1998). *The afro-centric idea.* Philadelphia, PA: Temple University Press.

Azibo, D.A. (Ed.) (1996). *African psychology in historical perspective and related commentary.* Trenton, New Jersey: Africa World Press, Inc.

Breton, M. (1990). Learning from social group work traditions. *Social Work with Groups,* 13(3), 21-34.

Byrne, D. (1971). *The attraction paradigm.* New York: Academic Press.

Caldwell, L.D. & White, J.L. (2001). African-centered therapeutic and counseling interventions for African American males. In G. Brooks & G. Good (Eds.), *A new handbook of counseling and psychotherapy approaches for men.* San Francisco: Jossey-Bass.

Chestang, L. (1976). The black family and black culture: A study in coping. In M. Sotomayer (Ed.), *Cross-cultural perspectives in social work practice and education.* Houston, TX: University of Houston Graduate School of Social Work.

Collins, L. (2003). The lost art of group work in camping. *Social Work with Groups,* 26(4), 21-41.

Cross, W., Parham, T., & Helms, J. (1985). Nigrescence revisited: Theory and research. In R. Jones (Ed.), *Advances in Black Psychology,* 81-98. New York: Harper & Row.

Dubois, W.E.B. (1903). *The souls of black folks.* New York: Penguin Books.

Erikson, E.H. (1968). *Identity, youth and crisis.* New York: Norton Press.

Fagan, J. & Wilkerson, D. (1998). Social contexts and functions of adolescent violence. In D.S. Elliott, B.A. Hamburg, & K.R. Williams (Eds.), *Violence In American Schools: A new perspective* (pp. 55-93). New York: Cambridge University Press

Gentry, M.E. (1984). Developments in activity analysis: Recreation and group work revisited. *Social Work with Groups,* 7(1), 35-44.

Gordon, M. (1964). *Assimilation in American life.* New York: Oxford University Press.

Green, J.W. (1982). *Cultural awareness in the human services.* Englewood Cliffs, NJ: Prentice-Hall.

Halliday-Boykins, C., Schoenwald, S., & Letourneau, E. (2005). Caregiver-therapist ethnic similarity predicts youth outcomes from an empirically based treatment. *Journal of Consulting and Clinical Psychology,* 73(5), 808-818.

Hare, N. & Hare, J. (1985). *Bringing the black boy to manhood: The passage.* San Francisco, CA: Black Think Tank.

Healey, J.F. (1995). *Race, ethnicity, gender, and class: The sociology of group conflict and change.* Thousand Oaks, CA: Forge Press.

Hill, J.P. & Lynch, M.E. (1983). The intensification of gender-related role expectations during early adolescence. In J. Brooks-Gunn & A.C. Petersen (Eds.), *Girls at puberty: Biological and psychological perspectives* (pp. 201-228). New York: Plenum Press.

Hutchinson. (1994). *The assassination of the black male Image.* Los Angeles, CA: Middle Passage Press.

Karenga, M. (1988). Black studies and the problematic paradigm: The philosophical dimension. *Journal of Black Studies,* 18, 395-414.

Karenga, M. (1989). *The African American holiday of Kwanzaa: A celebration of family, community & culture.* Los Angeles: University of Sankore Press.

Kroeber, A.L. & Kluckholm, C. (1952). *Culture: A critical review of concepts and definitions.* Cambridge, MA: Papers of the Peabody Museum No. 47.

Linton, R. (1945). *The cultural background of personality.* New York: Appleton-Century-Crofts.

Logan, S., Freeman, E., & McRoy, R. (1990). *Social work practice with black families: A culturally specific perspective.* White Plains, NY: Longman.

Logan, S. (2000). *The black family: Strengths, self-Help, and positive change.* Boulder, CO. Westview Press.

Michalski, J., Mishna, F., Worthington, C., & Cummings, R. (2003). A multi- method impact evaluation of a therapeutic summer camp program. *Child and Adolescent Social Work Journal,* 20(1), 53-76.

Mishna, F., Michalski, J., & Cummings, R. (2001). Camps as social work interventions: Returning to our roots. *Social Work with Groups,* 24(3/4), 153-171.

Nobles, W.W. (1984). Alienation, human transformation and adolescent drug use: Toward a reconceptualization of the problem. *Journal of Drug Issues,* 14(2), 243-252.

Ogbu, J.U. (1990). *Mentoring minority youth: A Framework.* New York: Columbia University, Teachers College, Institute for Urban and Minority Education.

Oliver, W. (1989). *Racial matters: The FBI's secret file on Black America, 1960-1972.* New York, NY: The Free Press.

Phillips, F.B. (1996). NTU Psychotherapy. Principles and processes. In Azibo, D.A. (Ed.), *African Psychology in Historical Perspective and Related Commentary* (pp. 83-99). Trenton, NJ: Africa World Press, Inc.

Redl, F. (1966). Psychopathological risks of camp life. In *When we deal with children: Selected writings* (pp. 440-451). New York, NY: The Free Press.

Robinson, T.L. & Howard-Hamilton, M.F. (2000). *The convergence of race, ethnicity, and gender: Multiple identities in counseling.* Upper Saddle River, NJ: Prentice Hall.

Rodney, H.E. & Mupier, R. (1999). Behavioral differences between African-American male adolescents with biological fathers and those without biological fathers in the house. *Journal of Black Studies,* 30(1), 45-61.

Rodney, H.E., Tachia, H.R., & Rodney, L.W. (1999). The home environment and delinquency: A study of African American adolescents. *Families in Society,* 80:551– 559.

Schiele, J.H. (2000). *Human services and the afro-centric paradigm.* Binghampton, NY: The Haworth Press.

Schwartz, W. (1960a). Camping. In T. Berman-Rossi (Ed.), *Social Work: The collected writings of William Schwartz* (pp. 419-426). (1994). Itasca, IL: F.E. Peacock Publishers.

Singer, M., Anglin, T.M., Song, L., & Lunghofer, L. (1995). Adolescents' exposure to violence and associated symptoms of psychological trauma. *Journal of the American Medical Association,* 273, 477-482.

Spencer, M.B. (1990). Development of minority children: An introduction. *Child Development,* 61, 267-269.

Spencer, M.B. & Markstrom-Adams, C. (1990). Identity processes among racial and ethnic minority children in America. *Child Development,* 61, 290-310.

Stevenson, H. (1994). Validation of the scale of racial socialization for African American adolescents: Steps toward multi-dimensionality. *Journal of Black Psychology,* 20(4), 445-468.

Sue, S., Fujino, D.c., Hu, L., Takeuchi, D.T., & Zane, N. (1991). Community mental health services for ethnic minority groups: A test of the cultural responsiveness hypothesis. *Journal of Consulting and Clinical Psychology, 59*, 533-540.

U.S. Department of Health and Human Services. (2001). *Mental health: Culture, race, and ethnicity/A supplement to mental health: A report to the Surgeon General.* Rockville, MD: Office of the Surgeon General.

Utsey, S.O., Howard, A., & Williams, O. (2003). Therapeutic group mentoring with African-American male adolescents. *Journal of Mental Health Counseling, 25,* 126-139.

Washington, G., Johnson, T., Jones, J., & Langs S. (2007). African-American boys in relative care: A culturally centered group mentoring approach. *Social Work with Groups, 30*(1), 45-69.

Willie, C.V. (1979). The inclining significance of race in the caste and class controvery, 10-15. Dix Hills, NY: General Hall Publishers.

Wilson, W.J. (1978). The declining significance of race revisited but not revised. *Society,* 11-21.

Wilson, W.F. (1987). *The truly disadvantaged: The inner city, the underclass, and public policy.* Chicago: University of Chicago Press.

Woodson, C.G. (1933). *The miseducation of the Negro.* Washington, DC: Associated Publishers.

Mental Health Issues and Psychotropic Medication: Current Applications for Children and Adolescents in Residential Treatment

Julie Worley, FNP, PMHNP

INTRODUCTION

Mental illness is a significant problem for many adolescents and their families. According to the Surgeon General's Report on Mental Health (1999), one in five children and youth have a diagnosable mental health, emotional, or behavioral disorder. The Center for Mental Health Services (Friedman et al., 1998) reports that one child out of every 33 experiences an episode of depression and that the same is true for one out of every eight adolescents. Further, children and youth who experience depression are at risk of experiencing a second episode within five years. Suicide is the sixth leading cause of death among juveniles between 5 and 14, and the third leading cause of death for youth between 15 and 24 (AACAP, 1997).

Although these statistics for the general population are sobering, the proportion of juveniles with serious mental health disorders is even greater among those in state's custody (Cocozza & Skowyra, April, 2000). As a result, expert estimates place the rate of juveniles with mental health disorders in the juvenile justice system at approximately 50%, (Friedman et al., 1996) and the rate of those with SMHD or SED at in excess of twenty per cent (Otto et al., 1992).

BIOCHEMISTRY, MENTAL ILLNESS, AND MEDICATION

The presence of so many youth with mental health issues in residential settings requires active, careful medical management. Frequently juveniles have been confined to residential settings for reasons such as chronic truancy, fighting, running away, substance abuse, and other illegal activities. Often their mental health issues have contributed to these problem behaviors.

In many cases mental illness is thought to be related to a chemical imbalance in the brain with alterations in neurotransmitter levels. These imbalances can be hereditary or genetic in nature. These are medical conditions similar to high blood pressure and diabetes, which are also chemical imbalances and run in families. Often we are seeing or recognizing these mental illnesses at earlier ages. Conversely, we also know that traumatic events can in some instances trigger or change the chemical balance in a persons brain. This could cause or create a mental illness such as Post Traumatic Stress Disorder (PTSD) or Major Depressive Disorder (MDD). In some cases trauma can trigger a predisposed mental illness such as Bipolar Disorder. It could also be theorized that a person may be genetically predisposed to developing depression or anxiety if they are exposed to trauma, but if they are not, they may not develop such an illness.

Children in residential settings often come from homes that are unstable, disruptive, neglectful or violent. Often there is a family history of mental illness in the immediate family members of the child in residential care. However, many children that are in residential settings come from single parent homes, are in foster care, or do not have contact with one or more of their parents so their family psychiatric history is completely or partially unknown.

BIPOLAR DISORDER

Bipolar disorder is a common diagnosis among children in residential placement. Patients with bipolar I disorder have experienced at least one episode of mania and may have experienced episodes of mixed, hypomanic or depressed states as well (American Psychiatric Association (APA) 2002).

According to the American Psychiatric Association Practice Guidelines, the prevalence of childhood bipolar disorder ranges from 1% of the general population meeting specific criteria to 5.7% meeting more generalized nonspecific criteria such as Bipolar NOS (American Psychiatric Association Practice Guidelines, 2002). A diagnosis of Bipolar NOS or Not Otherwise Specified is made when a person has bipolar symptoms but they do not meet the criteria for either Bipolar I or II. Consistent with the data on the prevalence of mental illness among adolescents in the juvenile justice system, it can be theorized that the incidence of bipolar disorder in residential treatment placements is higher than the general population. In fact, many children in residential settings do report a family member that also has bipolar disorder, previously called manic depression. Bipolar disorder is characterized by mood swings, periods of depression alternating with mind racing, agitation, increased energy level or hyperness, talking fast, needing less sleep, anger outbursts, and impulsivity. All these symptoms can lead to children having disrupted family relationships, problems with authority, acting out, and self-medicating with illegal substances. Often children with bipolar disorder have more mixed states, meaning they rapidly switch from one mood to another. In many cases in both children and adults there may be very few if any incidences of full blown mania but instead there may be what is termed hypomania as defined above, which is a less severe form of mania.

There are many misconceptions about bipolar disorder, some of which are relics of an evolving understanding. Currently it is seen more as a spectrum disorder with most patients falling on the milder or less severe side of the spectrum. This can be one reason why it is so frequently misdiagnosed. It is a fallacy that all people with bipolar disorder go from being extremely happy to being extremely depressed. In most cases people with bipolar disorder are not happy when manic or hypomanic, they may have more energy but it is usually not a good energy. Instead it is an agitated, restless, anxious state where they cannot concentrate and can't focus and become easily irritable and angry. Some patients with bipolar disorder go from feeling depressed to being on top the world and feeling they are invincible and can do anything. This, however, is not the conditions most common manifestation. Likewise, some of the more extreme behaviors generally believed to be associated with bipolar disorder are fairly rare. People going on extreme buying sprees, dressing totally out of character, acting out sexually, and essentially acting like a completely different person is not as commonly seen.

Bipolar disorder can sometimes occur with the presence of psychotic features. These are hallucinations, delusions, and paranoia. The psychotic symptoms can occur in either phase of the bipolar disorder but more commonly occur in the manic or hypomanic phase, especially with little sleep. It is not uncommon for youth who have bipolar disorder to experience either visual or auditory hallucinations.

Currently there are no separate criteria for diagnosing childhood bipolar disorder but we do know that it is often characterized by more rapidly changing moods or mixed states. The American Psychiatric Association Practice Guidelines state that:

> Although the DSM-IV criteria are used to diagnose bipolar disorder in children and adolescents, the clinical features of childhood bipolar disorder differ from bipolar disorder in adults. Children with bipolar disorder often have mixed manic, rapid cycling, and psychosis. (American Psychiatric Association, 2002)

According to the Child and Adolescent Bipolar Foundation, behaviors reported by parents in children diagnosed with bipolar disorder *may* include:

- an expansive or irritable mood
- extreme sadness or lack of interest in play
- rapidly changing moods lasting a few hours to a few days
- explosive, lengthy, and often destructive rages
- separation anxiety
- defiance of authority
- hyperactivity, agitation, and distractibility
- sleeping little or, alternatively, sleeping too much
- bed wetting and night terrors
- strong and frequent cravings, often for carbohydrates and sweets
- excessive involvement in multiple projects and activities
- impaired judgment, impulsivity, racing thoughts, and pressure to keep talking
- dare-devil behaviors (such as jumping out of moving cars or off roofs)
- inappropriate or precocious sexual behavior
- delusions and hallucinations
- grandiose belief in own abilities that defy the laws of logic (ability to fly, for example) (Child and Adolescent Bipolar Foundation, 2002).

Again, genetics plays a role in bipolar disorder. The Child and Adolescent Bipolar Foundation offers the following observation:

The family trees of many children who develop early-onset bipolar disorder include individuals who suffered from substance abuse and/or mood disorders (often undiagnosed). Also among their relatives are found highly-accomplished, creative, and extremely successful individuals in business, politics, and the arts.

- For the general population, a conservative estimate of an individual's risk of having full-blown bipolar disorder is 1 percent. Disorders in the bipolar spectrum may affect 4-6%.
- When one parent has bipolar disorder, the risk to each child is 15-30%.
- When both parents have bipolar disorder, the risk increases to 50-75%.
- The risk in siblings and fraternal twins is 15-25%.
- The risk in identical twins is approximately 70%.

In every generation since World War II, there is a higher incidence and an earlier age of onset of bipolar disorder and depression. On average, children with bipolar disorder experience their first episode of illness 10 years earlier than their parents' generation did. The reason for this is unknown. (Child and Adolescent Bipolar Foundation, 2002)

Medications used to treat bipolar disorder include mood stabilizers and atypical neuroleptics. In most cases, mood stabilizers are the first line treatment. There are five medications in this drug class; Lithium, Depakote, Tegretol, Trileptal, and Lamictal. In the recent past Topamax was also used routinely and long ago Neurontin was also used but studies have not proven their effectiveness so they are no longer considered mood stabilizers. Currently the only mood stabilizer that is approved by the Food and Drug Administration (FDA) for children is Depakote. Regardless, other medications are routinely used and considered within the standard of care in treating childhood bipolar disorder.

In psychiatry medications that are not FDA approved for certain psychiatric uses or not in children are routinely used and this is called "off label" use. The reason that many drugs in psychiatry do not have certain FDA approvals or indications is often a financial issue on the part of drug companies that have chosen not to pay the millions of dollars to get another FDA approval. In other cases a medication may be available in a generic form, so there is no motivation for a drug company to seek further FDA approvals when they cannot benefit financially or recoup the cost of the research that has to be done to get additional indications. As for the mood stabilizers, all but Lithium are also seizure medications or anticonvulsants, that are FDA approved for seizures in children, so their safety has already been determined in children. Not all seizure medications work for bipolar disorder. The reason that the mood stabilizers also treat seizures is that some of the same neurotransmitters that play a role in mood stabilization also regulate seizure activity. Lithium is the only mood stabilizer that is not an anticonvulsant. It is, in fact, a salt and is in a drug class of its own.

Side effects can be issues with medications used to treat bipolar disorder. In the mood stabilizer class lithium, depakote, and tegretal can all cause weight gain. Blood work must also be done regularly on patients taking lithium, depakote, and tegretal and initially with trileptal. Drowsiness can also occur with lithium, depakote and tegretol and occasionally with trileptal. Lamictal does not have the weight gain or drowsiness side effect and lab work does not need to be done. There is a rare very serious sensitivity rash associated with lamictal. For this reason lamictal is started at a very low dose and gradually increased so that there is less of a chance of the rash occurring. If a rash does occur, the medication has to be stopped immediately and the patient will not be able to continue to take it. The rash is very rare but is slightly more common to occur in children than adults.

Recently atypical neuroleptic medications have gotten FDA approval to treat bipolar disorder. None of these medications are FDA approved to treat bipolar disorder in children, however, they are routinely used. Neuroleptics, once called antipsychotics, were initially made in the 1950s such as haldol and thorazine. In the 1990s a newer class of medications was derived from this older class called atypical neuroleptics, sometimes also referred to as second generation antipsychotics (SGAs). For the purpose of this article, they will be referred to as atypical neuroleptics. Rarely are the older neuroleptics used today, especially in children due to side effects, except when cost is an issue and occasionally they are used as add on medication to the atypical neuroleptics in severe cases. The cost of the older neuroleptics would average around $40 a month whereas the atypical neuroleptics cost on average from $200 to

$600 per month depending on the dosage. Atypical neuroleptics include Risperdal, Seroquel, Zyprexa, Geodon, and Abilify. Clozaril is another medication that is also considered an atypical neuroleptic but it is not routinely used in children because but it is reserved for severe psychotic cases that have not responded to any other treatment due to the fact that is associated with a rare blood disorder. Initially these drugs were FDA approved to treat bipolar mania but some newer studies are showing they may help the depression phase as well. Symbiax is a combination drug of Zyprexa and Prozac and it is FDA approved for bipolar depression. Atypical neuroleptics work by blocking dopamine, a neurotransmitter in the brain. Increased dopamine is associated with psychotic symptoms such as hallucinations, delusions and paranoia. We do not fully understand how but dopamine also plays a role in other symptoms such as depression, anger, preoccupation, obsessiveness, and other behavior disturbances. As previously stated, none of the atypical neuroleptics are FDA approved to treat bipolar disorder in children under age 18. However Risperdal did just get FDA approval to treat irritability in children over age five with Autism, so some safety for this class being used in children has been established and these drugs have been used extensively to treat children.

The neuroleptic drug class could be considered the "strongest" psychiatric medications available and initially were used only to treat psychotic illnesses such as schizophrenia. Today however, in addition to treating psychosis and bipolar disorder, they are commonly used "off label" to treat other conditions such as Obsessive Compulsive Disorder (OCD), treatment resistant depression, and for symptoms such as anger, disruptive behavior, severe PTSD symptoms, and preoccupied thinking.

This class of medication can also be associated with significant side effects. Although much less common than their ancestors, atypical neuroleptics can cause involuntary muscle movements called extrapyramidal symptoms (EPS). Weight gain can be very problematic in this drug class, found most significant in Zyprexa and least significant in Abilify and Geodon. The weight gain is related to increased appetite and a decrease in the sensation of fullness. When weight gain occurs and there is a genetic predisposition for diabetes, blood glucose levels can rise, so periodic monitoring of blood sugar as well as cholesterol is necessary to be monitored in persons taking this drug class. Sedation occurs with Zyprexa, Seroquel, and Risperdal is varying degrees with each person due to saturation of histamine receptors in the brain. The sedation side effect is often desirable as many people with bipolar disorder have problems sleeping although this can be problematic if residual daytime drowsiness results. Geodon and Abilify are least likely to cause sedation. Abilify can have a rare side effect of akithesia, which is a type of restlessness. Abilify is the newest in this drug class and probably has the most favorable side effect profile but one issue with it is cost, often being double of the other atypical neuroleptics.

Many times children in residential placement are in state's custody and therefore on state health insurance plans, which often have formularies listing preferred drugs they will cover. In some states for instance, a provider must first prescribe at least one or more of the less expensive medication on their formulary before the state will pay for the more expensive medication.

While treating patients with the least number of medications is always preferable, it has been estimated that up to 60-70% of people with bipolar disorder will require both classes of medications, mood stabilizers and atypical neuroleptics in order to adequately treat their symptoms. As previously stated, in the past mood stabilizers were the first line treatment for bipolar disorder, but now with the atypical neuroleptics getting FDA approval for treating some of the symptoms of bipolar disorder, some providers are using them for first line treatment. Treatment regimes will vary from provider to provider. Often which medication is chosen initially is determined by the type or severity of the symptoms that the patient presents with.

Bipolar disorder is a medical illness that must be treated long term with medication. As with high blood pressure or diabetes where a person cannot change their blood pressure or blood sugar level by trying, the same is true with bipolar disorder. Medication is a permanent necessity. Unlike most other mental illnesses other than psychosis, counseling alone cannot treat this disorder. People with bipolar disorder have higher rates of suicide, and higher incidences of instability with employment and relationships, which worsen if they are not on medication. There is a tendency for people with bipolar disorder, similar to most mental illnesses to at some point begin to think that they no longer need their medication or to get tired of having to take medication and then stop it. This will inevitably result in problems. Children and teenagers often do not want to take medication and they should be closely monitored by parents to be sure they are taking their medication. While this is not as much of an issue in residential settings, teenagers do have certain rights to refuse medication. Some jurisdictions allow children who have reached a specified age (often around 15) to choose which medications they will and will not take. When a teenager refuses to take medication for bipolar disorder there can be devastating consequences. This can also be an issue if a child is released back to the custody of parents or guardians who do not believe in the child taking psychotropic medications. Education and support are keys to medication compliance.

MAJOR DEPRESSIVE DISORDER

Major Depressive Disorder (MDD) Another common diagnosis among children in residential placement. Again, this disorder can be genetic and run in families. In addition traumatic events such as a death or abuse can also trigger depression. However, a determination needs to be made on what is a normal grief reaction or normal sadness versus something that would be classified as a medical condition and require medication. Many children in residential placement may be sad and upset about their situation or their past but this does not necessarily mean that they need medication. The severity of the symptoms and how they are affecting their everyday life need to be carefully explored before the use of medication should be considered. Studies have shown that in children counseling can be as effective as medication in treating most cases of depression so this should most always be the first line treatment for depression in children.

Another consideration in treating childhood depression is that there can be adverse reactions to antidepressants in children. Recently the FDA mandated a black box warning on all Selective Seratonin Reuptake Inhibitor (SSRI) antidepressants, which is the most widely used antidepressant class today. These medications include Prozac, Zoloft, Paxil, Lexapro, and Celexa. The issue of using SSRIs to treat children is a controversial issue. Since their use, the suicide rate in children has decreased however there have been several highly publicized cases of children committing suicide after having taken antidepressants.

The reasons that a person may commit suicide after being placed on an antidepressant are complex. In some cases, a person may have been so severely depressed before starting the medication that the medication does not have time to work. There is usually a three-week time frame before the medication will begin to work and then often it will require that the dosage be gradually increased to achieve an optimal effect. In other cases, a person may have already been suicidal before starting on the medication and are acting out on a plan that they already had unrelated to the antidepressant use. In other cases a person may be misdiagnosed with depression and in actuality have a different chemical imbalance such as bipolar disorder. Antidepressants can trigger a manic episode or cause a person with bipolar disorder to become more irritable and agitated and thus could lead to a suicide attempt. Even in people that do not have bipolar disorder, in some cases antidepressants can cause a person to experience side effects of restlessness and irritability and this may be magnified in some children. All children placed on antidepressants need to be closely monitored for any worsening symptoms or suicidal thoughts.

While it may seem best for children not to be on antidepressants due to the possible side effects or risks, depression is a real and debilitating condition for many children and does often respond well to medication. Children with severe depression may experience overwhelming sadness, hopelessness, crying, irritability, poor sleep and poor self esteem which all can lead to suicidal thoughts. As previously stated a very important fact remains that since antidepressants have been prescribed for children, the suicide rate in children has declined and there is evidence that using antidepressants in children and adults does decrease the incidence of suicide. If a child has persistent severe symptoms of depression that does not respond to counseling, antidepressants need to be considered.

POST-TRAUMATIC STRESS DISORDER

Another common diagnosis in children in residential placement is Post-Traumatic Stress Disorder (PTSD). This can result from any real or perceived threat to the child. Many children in residential settings have a history of physical or sexual abuse. Some adolescents have also been raped. Witnessing violence such as domestic abuse is also common and can lead to symptoms of PTSD. Symptoms of PTSD include flashbacks and nightmares about the traumatic event. In addition to therapy, antidepressants are often used to treat persistent and severe symptoms of PTSD. In more severe cases, atypical neuroleptics may be prescribed.

ANXIETY DISORDERS

Anxiety is a common complaint in adolescents in residential placement. This can occur as a symptom in depression or PTSD but can also rarely be Generalized Anxiety Disorder (GAD). This finding needs to be carefully examined and considered in children as well as adults in order to ascertain the underlying cause. Bipolar disorder always needs to be ruled out because people in manic or hypomanic states will often describe how they feel as anxious. Counseling to treat the underlying cause of anxiety unrelated to bipolar disorder is preferred to medication in children. SSRI antidepressants are FDA approved to treat anxiety so this may be an option in some cases but as stated before there are risks involved. Since many adolescents in residential placement have substance abuse issues, complaining of anxiety may indicate a drug seeking behavior. Controlled drugs, which are drugs that are determined to cause dependence or tolerance should not be routinely used in children, especially if there is a substance abuse history. Benzodiazapines, often referred to as "nerve pills" such as xanax, ativan, klonopin, and valium are generally not recommended for this population.

ATTENTION DEFICIT HYPERACTIVITY DISORDER

Another diagnosis that children in residential placement present with or are diagnosed with is Attention Deficit Disorder (ADHD), which can occur with or without hyperactivity. This needs to be carefully analyzed and considered because this is frequently a misdiagnosis for bipolar disorder. In addition there is a higher incidence of ADHD in people with bipolar disorder. Many symptoms of ADHD such as distractibility, inability to concentrate, impulsivity, and irritability mimic those of bipolar disorder. In general, the symptoms are magnified in bipolar disorder and the medications normally used to treat ADHD will either not work or will make a person with bipolar disorder worse. The medications used to treat ADHD are either Strattera, which increases norepinephrine levels similar to that of the antidepressant wellbutrin or stimulants, which are amphetamines such as Ritalin, Adderall, and Concerta. Since antidepressants can make people with bipolar disorder or plain depression worse caution needs to be taken when prescribing Strattera for children that may have bipolar disorder but are misdiagnosed with ADHD. Stimulants can also make some children worse as far as more aggressive or hostile. If a child has both diagnosis of bipolar disorder and ADHD, the general consensus is to treat the bipolar disorder and this usually leads to an improvement in all symptoms including ADHD. Considering the high incidence of substance abuse among teenagers in residential placement, prescribing a highly controlled substance such as stimulants is not generally recommended however there is some controversy in this area. Some studies have shown that people with symptoms of ADHD that are treated with stimulants have a lower incidence of substance abuse. However, most clinicians would be reluctant to prescribe stimulants to teenagers in residential placement that have a history of substance abuse. It is estimated that the diversion rate or rate of someone other than the patient taking the stimulant medication prescribed in homes is about 40%. This would occur if the parents took the child's medication and used it as speed or if the child gave or sold the medication to friends, etc. Since the majority of these children will eventually leave placement and may be returning to homes where there is a history of substance abuse this is also a factor in why prescribing stimulants to this population is not common.

All children in residential placement need to have a psychological evaluation in order to determine if a mental illness exists and if they should be referred for medication management. Since the placement in a residential setting in and of itself is traumatic and stressful to children, counseling is always advisable. If it is discovered that counseling alone is not alleviating more severe mental health illness this indicates a referral for medication management. Medications need to be used cautiously in children and closely monitored, but when indicated, in many cases they are used successfully and result in improvement to the child's overall mental health.

CONCLUSION

The presence of a high proportion of juveniles with severe mental health conditions makes accurate diagnosis and careful medication management critical components of effective adolescent residential treatment. Recent developments of new medications and applications of pre-existing medications have made treatment increasingly successful. This paper summarizes the major mental illnesses most commonly encountered in adolescent residential treatment, then describes the medications often used to treat them. Although the paper does not constitute medical advice, it is offered to facilitate the understanding of the many non-medical practitioners in the mental health field.

REFERENCES

American Academy of Child and Adolescent Psychiatry. (1997). Facts for Families: Teen Suicide. (Available online: http://www.aacap.org/page.ww?section= Facts%20for%20Families&name=Teen%20Suicide).

American Psychiatric Association. (1994). *Diagnostic and Statistical Manual of Mental Disorders (4th ed.)*. Washington DC: American Psychiatric Press.

American Psychiatric Association, *Practice Guidelines Second Edition*. (2002). Retrieved March 18, 2007 from http://www.psych.org/psych_pract/treatg/pg/Bipolar2ePG_05-15-06.pdf

Center for Mental Health Services. (1998).

Child and Adolescent Bipolar Foundation. (2002). *About Pediatric Bipolar Disorder*. (Available online: http://www.bpkids.org/site/PageServer?pagename=lrn_about).

Cocozza, J.J., & Skowya, K.R. (2000). Youth with Mental Disorders: Issues and Emerging Responses. *Juvenile Justice*, VII(1), 3-13.

Freidman, R.M., Katz-Leavy, J.W., Mandershied, R.W., & Sandheimer, D.L. (1996). Prevalence of serious emotional disturbances in children and adolescents. In *Mental Health, United States*, (Ed.) R.W. Mandersheid and M.A. Sonnerschein. Washington, DC: U.S. Department of Health and Human Services, Substance Abuse and Mental Health Services Administration, Center for Mental Health Services, pp. 71-89.

Otto, R.K., Greenstein, J.J., Johnson, M.K., & Friedman, R.M. (1992). Prevalence of mental disorders among youth in the juvenile justice system. *In Responding to the Mental Health Needs of Youth in the Juvenile Justice System* (JJ. Cocozza, Ed.)

Seattle, WA: The National Coalition for the Mentally Ill in the Criminal Justice System.

US Office of the Surgeon General. (1999). Mental Health: A Report of the Surgeon General. (Available online: http://www.surgeongeneral.gov/library/mentalhealth/home.html).

Mentoring and Other Adult Involvement with Juveniles in Treatment: Do They Decrease the Probability of Elopement?

Michael L. Burford, MSSW
William R. Nugent, PhD
John Wodarski, PhD

INTRODUCTION

Runaway youth are a familiar problem to those who work in congregate care social service organizations. Some adolescents run away despite best efforts of professional and line staff at preventing such risky behavior. In discussing the issue, Deni (1990) reports that "Children running away . . . are not a new problem, but today children are running in increasing numbers" (p. 1).

Adolescents who elope from their caretakers place themselves at risk in that they must find food and safe shelter (Kidd, 2003; Baker, McKay, Lynn, Schlange, and Auville, 2003), often engage in prostitution, have promiscuous sex with friends, and use drugs (Greene, Ennett, and Ringwalt, 1999; Hagan and McCarthy, 1997). Such behaviors increase probability of getting diseases such as AIDS and hepatitis (Booth, Zhang, and Kwiatkowski, 1999; Rotheram-Borus, Koopman, and Ehrhardt, 1991). Further, running away interrupts or terminates progress toward developing skills useful in resolving troublesome issues that may have contributed to the running behavior (Abbey, Nicholas, and Bieber, 1997), and that could ultimately lead to reunification with loved ones. Greene, Ringwalt, and Iachen (1997) further explain that "Because runaway adolescents typically lack the skills and education necessary to obtain and maintain gainful employment, they often are forced into prostitution, drug dealing, and other criminal behavior to survive."

LITERATURE REVIEW

Little information is found regarding adolescents who run away from residential congregate care treatment centers. In her study of runners from a runaway shelter, Roe (2000) says that "Much research has been conducted to explain why adolescents run away from home; yet little information exists on why adolescents run from residential care in the child welfare system" (p. 6). Kashubeck, Pottebaum, and Read (1994) report that " . . . there are few published empirical studies exploring the phenomenon of elopement from psychiatric facilities" (p. 127).

While more work on residential care runaways is needed, some formal and published research has been done. As early as the 1970s, Levy (1972) explored running away from congregate care, concluding that it "is a complex of causes, types, impacts, meanings, staff reactions and management efforts" (p. 1). Kashubeck, Pottebaum, and Read (1994) report predictors of running behavior that include a prior history of running away, diagnosis of an affective disorder, having parental rights of both parents terminated (this variable alone was found to be insufficient as a predictor and is useful only in conjunction with other variables), a history of multiple residential setting changes, and difficulties with attachment and separation. Findings from a study by Abbey, Nicholas, and Bieber (1997) generally support the results of Kashubeck, Pottebaum, and Reads. However, while Kashubeck, Pottebaum, and Read (1994) did not find a significant relationship between running away and physical abuse or legal offenses, Abbey, Nicholas, and Bieber (1997) did find that "runners were more likely to have a history of physical abuse, both as perpetrator and victim, and to be offenders of property crimes" (p. 82).

In discussing the results of her study on runners from a residential care facility as compared to non-runners, Roe (2000) explains that: "Runners were proportionately more likely than non-runners to have been Caucasian, a victim of neglect, to not have been a victim of physical abuse, had their parent's parental rights terminated, had a history of drug abuse and have had a history of illegal activity. Runners were also proportionately more likely to have average physical health, be placed on observe or at-risk status by CEGU, had been prescribed psychotropic medication while detained and had poor relationships with staff" (p. 48).

According to Kidd (2003), several participants in his study on street youth "spoke of being moved numerous times to group and foster homes, being abused and trapped in environments in which people did not care about them" (p. 251). Kidd's study appears to support the importance kids place on feeling like someone cares about them; they seem to need at least one stable, nurturing relationship. Unfortunately, it appears that many kids do not have such relationships.

METHODS

Description of the Study

Does having someone actively involved (via off grounds passes) in their lives (as mentors, family members, or older friends) really make a difference in terms of whether an adolescent runs from a residential facility? The purpose of this study was to answer the question as to whether a relationship exists between running away and attending off grounds passes (such passes are an indicator of an actively involved adult).

It was believed that adolescents who have active, positive relationships (measured by frequency and duration of off grounds pass occurrences with the adolescent and the involved adult) with a dependable person would be less likely to run away (or will be absent shorter periods of time if they do run away). Hypothesis number one stated that as off grounds pass occurrences increase, frequency of runaways would decrease. Hypothesis number two stated that as the number of hours spent on off grounds passes increases, the frequency of runaways would decrease. Hypothesis number three stated that as off grounds pass occurrences increase, runaway hours would decrease. Hypothesis number four stated that as number of off grounds pass hours increases, runaway hours would decrease. Spearman's rho and linear regression were used to analyze data.

Data Collection

Case files of former clients who received services at a southern residential agency were used in this study. Data was collected from 200 closed case files of male and female clients who resided in any one of nine residential facilities belonging to the mental health treatment agency.

Files for this study dated from 1988 to 2005. The total population from which a sample size of 200 was pulled is 2,130. Files used for the sample were chosen at random.

Independent variables analyzed were length of stay in congregate care, type of permanency goal, availability and number of off grounds pass resources (whether such a resource exists for that particular client), number of actual off grounds passes that occurred, duration of off grounds passes (in cumulative hours), and number of off grounds passes approved by DCS that did not occur. This work also investigated links between running away and client demographics (age, sex, and ethnicity), adjudication (dependent and neglected or delinquent), history of drug abuse, spiritual/religious affiliation, and use of prescription psychoactive medications. Dependent variables were number of runaways and runaway hours.

RESULTS

Sample Characteristics

The client sample consisted of males (69.5%) and females (30.5%) between the ages of 10 and 19 years, with a mean age of 15.5 years (S. D. = 1.71). The sample showed an ethnic mix, with the predominant ethnicity represented being Caucasian (81.3%) and African American (16.1%). Latinos accounted for 2.1% and "other" was .5%. It also consisted of wards of the State, with 60.6% having been placed in State custody by the court system and adjudicated as being delinquent, and 39.4% as having been found to be dependent and neglected by their primary caregiver. Forty-six and a half percent of the sample had a record of being prescribed psycho-active medications, and 64.5 % had a history of abusing drugs (including alcohol). Forty-five and a half percent reported having religious or spiritual beliefs.

Concerning permanency resources, 47% of the sample had a goal of reunification with parent(s), nine percent had relative placement indicated, ten percent had foster care or adoption listed, 15% had independent living goals, and four percent had emancipation as a goal. The remaining 15% of the sample consisted of cases where no single permanency resource had been identified, meaning that several permanency options may have existed and the best would have been utilized as it became apparent based on developing information and opportunity.

The mean length of stay in residential care for subjects in the sample was 159 days, with a minimum of one day and a maximum of 797 days (S.D. = 149 days). One-hundred-twenty clients in the sample did not run away, 49 ran once, 18 ran twice, eight ran three times, three ran four times, one ran seven times and one ran seventeen times. Hours spent on runaway status had a mean of 93 hours (S.D. = 265.5), a minimum of 0 run hours and a maximum of 2,016 hours (this number was high as information from the file indicated the client ran away but was not removed from the census for an extended length of time, which precluded more recent policy concerning bed-holds and running away). The next highest number was 852. It was noted that 75% of all runners were absent 48 hours or less.

Regarding off grounds pass resources found in the sample, 44% did not have off grounds pass resources, 25% had one, 22% had two, seven percent had three, one percent had four, and .5% had five off ground pass resources. Off ground pass resource information existed for 198 subjects in the sample, with a mean of .96 (S.D. = 1.05). Of clients that went on off ground passes, 28% were taken by parents, six percent by relatives, .5% by volunteers, .5 percent by employees of The Department of Children's Services, seven percent by parents and relatives (each served as a resource and engaged in pass activity at different times), three percent by parents and a volunteer, two percent by a foster family, .5 % by parents and foster family, and three percent had multiple people of varying relationships that served as pass resources.

Forty-eight percent of the sample did not attend off grounds passes, twelve percent had one off grounds pass, five percent had two off grounds passes, five percent had three off grounds passes, and three percent had four off grounds passes. The mean for off grounds pass attendance was 4.40 (S.D. = 7.9), with a maximum number of off grounds passes for a case having been 44. Although the maximum number of off grounds pass hours was 4703, the mean was 157 hours with a standard deviation of 444.78. Two and a half percent of the sample had one instance of an off grounds pass resource that refused pass activity, and .5% (one case) had 14 instances of a resource that denied off grounds pass activity. Such neglected off grounds passes in the sample had a mean of .0950 (S.D. = 1.00). Five percent of the sample had off grounds passes denied once by authorities such as judges and State caseworkers, .5% had off grounds passes denied twice, and no record exists of off grounds passes having been denied more than twice for any case in the sample. Denied off grounds passes had a mean of .06 (S.D. = .29).

Missing Data

Missing data found in variables were as follows: age, 1%; sex, 1.5%; ethnicity, 3.5%; adjudication, 3.5%; length of stay in care, 1%; runaway absence measured in hours, 4%; permanency resource, 8.5%; number of off grounds pass resources, 1%; off grounds pass relationships, .5%; off grounds passes denied by authorities, .5%. The variables of number of runaways, off grounds passes attended, off grounds pass hours, off grounds passes declined by off grounds pass resource, age, religious/spiritual beliefs, and drug abuse had no missing data. As data were missing for some variables, a missing indicator variable was created for all variables where the number "one" was designated for a missing variable and "zero" was given for data that was not missing.

Simple Correlation

As variables in this study were not normally distributed, preventing the use of parametric methods. Therefore, Spearman's rho was used to determine correlations. P-values are converted into one tailed values because the research hypotheses are one directional, and to add power to the statistical tests of the correlations.

Table 1 shows that a negative correlation was found between number of runaways and number of off grounds passes attended, with a correlation coefficient of −.17 and a p-value of .01. The number of runaways was also negatively correlated with off grounds pass hours, with a correlation coefficient of −.16, and a p-value of .01. These results were consistent with the research hypotheses. Runaway hours had a negative correlation of −.18 and a p-value of .01 with number of off grounds passes attended. Runaway hours and off grounds pass hours were also negatively correlated, with a correlation coefficient of −.17 and a P-value of .01. These results were also consistent with the research hypotheses.

As discussed above, number of runaways and runaway hours were negatively correlated with number off grounds passes attended and off

TABLE 1. Correlations

			Runaway Incidences	Runaway Hours	Pass Frequency	Pass Hours
spearman's rho	runaway incidences	Correlation Coefficient	1.000	.961**	−.167*	−.155*
		sig. (2-tailed)	.	.000	.018	.028
		N		200	192	200	200
	runaway hours	Correlation Coefficient	.961**	1.000	−.177*	−.166*
		sig. (2-tailed)	.000	.	.014	.022
		N	192	192	192	192
	pass frequency	Correlation Coefficient	−.167*	−.177*	1.000	.961**
		sig. (2-tailed)	.018	.014	.	.000
		N	200	192	200	200
	pass hours	Correlation Coefficient	−.155*	−.166*	.961**	1.000
		sig. (2-tailed)	.028	.022	.000	.
		N	200	192	200	200

* Correlation is significant at the 0.05 level (2-tailed).
** Correlation is significant at the 0.01 level (2-tailed).

grounds pass hours, although these variables were only weakly correlated. However, a weak correlation and significant p-value could have been the result of artifacts. As such, regression analyses were needed to help establish whether a relationship existed between dependent variables and independent variables, controlling for possible confounding variables.

Multiple Linear Regression

Several covariates may have influenced the correlations between the independent and dependent variables. Multiple linear regression was used to control for the covariates of age, adjudication, and drug abuse. Age was controlled as it appeared reasonable that older adolescents may have been more likely to run away as they may have wanted autonomy and been less afraid of defying authority. Adjudication was controlled as delinquent adolescents may have been more prone than non-delinquents to defy authority and run away, especially considering they already had a history of using deficient problem solving skills. Drug abuse was also controlled as some clients may have run away to satisfy strong cravings to use drugs. Any or all of these covariates may have influenced the correlations between off grounds passes attended, off grounds pass hours, runaway frequency, and runaway hours.

Hypothesis One

Hypothesis one stated that as off grounds pass occurrences increase, runaway numbers would decrease. After controlling for age, adjudication, and drug abuse, the relationship between number of off grounds passes attended and runaway numbers was significant: $b = -.02$, $t = -2.05$, $p = .021$ (see Table 2). These results suggested that, after controlling for covariates, there was an inverse relationship between numbers of off grounds passes attended and number of runaways, and the relationship was in the predicted direction (as off grounds passes increased in frequency, runaways decreased). However, the change in number of runaways in relation to number of off grounds passes attended was small, as was the proportion of variance of number of runaways uniquely explained by number of off grounds passes, .021 (or 2.1%).

TABLE 2. Coefficients

Variables	B	t	Sig
Number of passes and number of runaway occurrences	−.02	−2.05	.021
Number of pass hours and number of runaway occurrences	.000	−1.4	.09
Number of passes and number of runaway hours	−3.43	−1.75	.04
Number of pass hours and number of runaway hours	−.04	−1.11	.135

Hypothesis Two

Hypothesis two was not supported, as the relationship between off grounds pass hours and runaway frequency was non-significant: $b = .000$, $t = -1.4$, $p = .09$. These results were not consistent with the hypothesis of a relationship between number of off grounds pass hours and runaway frequency.

Hypothesis Three

The relationship between number of off grounds passes attended and runaway hours, controlling for covariates, was significant: $b = -3.43$, $t = -1.75$, $p = .04$, and the proportion of variance of runaway hours uniquely explained by number of off grounds passes was .016. Number of off grounds passes appeared, in this sample, to be related to runaway hours. These results supported the research hypothesis.

Hypothesis Four

The relationship between off grounds pass hours and runaway hours, controlling for covariates, was non-significant: $b = -.04$, $t = -1.11$, $p = .135$. These findings did not support the hypothesis that increased off grounds pass hours would be negatively associated with runaway hours.

DISCUSSION

Reviewing the data and analysis, correlations suggested that frequency of off grounds passes and length of time, measured in hours, spent on off grounds passes were negatively related to runaway frequency and runaway hours. However, when the covariates of age, adjudication and drug abuse were controlled, there appeared to only be a relationship between number of off grounds passes attended and runaway incidences, and between number of off grounds passes attended and runaway hours. As frequency of off grounds passes increased, runaway frequency and duration decreased. No relationship was found between hours spent engaged in off grounds pass activity and runaway frequency and duration. As such, it was reasonably concluded that there may be a relationship between involvement of a pass resource, be it parent, relative, or volunteer, and runaway occurrences.

Limitations

One limitation concerns the generalizability of this study sample to the national runaway population. While this study used a sample of client charts from eight congregate care homes, caution is advised in inferring generalizations as these homes are all part of the same agency, and are not necessarily representative of other populations. Whitbeck and Hoyt (1999) concur, pointing out that "Because research reports tend to be bound to single shelters or cities, we cannot make generalizations about characteristics of runaway and homeless youth with great confidence" (p. 7). Because this work suggested that off grounds pass activity with an involved adult is related to practices of running away, further studies considering these variables and using data from other agencies and cities are needed.

Another limitation is the measurement of adult involvement. This work has defined adult involvement as taking a client on an off grounds pass. It appears reasonable that there are other ways that adults may be involved in a client's care, excluding engaging in off grounds pass activity. Further, it is known what role the adults may have played in their interactions with the youths. Some may have served as mentors, some may have been family members, and some older friends or extended family. Caution must be taken in assuming adult involvement is limited to taking clients on off grounds passes; simply visiting clients may be meaningful to clients in such a way as to influence behavioral changes.

Further limitations include issues of consistency in the way data were originally recorded. Records were produced by different employees that worked with the clients, which may reflect variation in the way data were recorded. Also, as some client files used in this study date back 17 years, records reflect that recording methods and policies used by staff to record information have changed numerous times. While every effort was made to maintain integrity and consistency when collecting data, it is possible that differences in recording methods and policies impact findings in this work.

Further, other variables that have not been identified or tested in this paper could play a role in running away, and may potentially show that no relationship exists between the dependent and independent variables.

CONCLUSION

Running away from a residential treatment center continues to be a serious problem for adolescents, their families, helping professionals, and the community. Whitbeck and Hoyt (1999) caution that adolescents who run away may " . . . progressively become entrapped by the consequences of their own behaviors. The accumulation of negative chains of events diminishes opportunities for change" (p. 12). They go on to state that "As the accumulation of negative experiences grows, options narrow, doors close" (p. 12).

In searching for variables that may impact running away from residential treatment centers, this study found a weak but statistically significant relationship between frequency of off grounds passes and runaway incidences, and between frequency of passes and hours spent on the run. There did not appear to be a relationship between number of hours spent on passes and frequency of runs, or between number of hours spent on passes and number of hours spent on the run. Further research is needed to substantiate these outcomes.

NOTE

The authors would like to acknowledge contributions made by David Dupper, PhD, at the College of Social Work, The University of Tennessee.

REFERENCES

Abbey, A. A., Nicholas, K. B., & Bieber, S. L. (1997). Predicting runaways upon admission to an adolescent treatment center. *Residential Treatment for Children and Youth, 15*, (2), 73-85.

Baker, A. J., McKay, M. M., Lynn, C. J., Schlange, H., & Auville, A. (2003). Recidivism at a shelter for adolescents: First-time versus repeat runaways. *Social Work Research, 27*, (2), 84-93.

Booth, R. E., Zhang, Y., & Kwiatkowski, C. F. (1999). The challenge of changing drug and sex risk behaviors of runaway and homeless adolescents. *Child Abuse and Neglect, 23*, 1295-1306.

Deni, J. R. (1990). Children and running away. *School Psychology Review, 19*, (2), 253-254.

Greene, J. M., Ennett, S. T., & Ringwalt, C. L. (1999). Prevalence and correlates of survival sex among runaway and homeless youth. *American Journal of Public Health, 89*, 1406-1409.

Greene, J. M., Ringwalt, C. L., & Iachen, R. (1997). Shelters for runaway and homeless youths: Capacity and occupancy. *Child Welfare, 76*, 549-561.

Hagen, J., & McCarthy, B. (1997). *Mean streets: Youth crime and homelessness.* Cambridge, UK: Cambridge University Press.

Kashubeck, S., Pottenbaum, S. M., & Read, N. O. (1994). Predicting elopement from residential treatment centers. *American Journal of Orthopsychiatry, 64*, (1), 126-135.

Kidd, S. A. (2003). Street Youth: Coping and Interventions. *Child and Adolescent Social Work Journal, 20*, (4), 235-261.

Levy, E. Z. (1972). Some thoughts about patients who run away from residential treatment and the staff they leave behind. *The Psychiatric Quarterly, 46*, (1), 1-21.

Rotheram-Borus, M. J., Koopman, C., & Ehrhardt, A. A. (1991). Homeless youths and HIV infection. *American Psychologist, 46*, 1188-1198.

Roe, E. J. (2000). Identifying factors associated with runaway behavior in adolescents placed in residential care in the child welfare system. Unpublished master's thesis, California State University, Long Beach.

Whitbeck, L. B., & Hoyt, D. R. (1999). *Nowhere to Grow.* New York, NY: Aldine De Gruyter.

Residential Treatment of Substance Abusing Adolescents: Trends in the Post-Managed Care Era

Samuel A. MacMaster, PhD
Rodney A. Ellis, PhD, CMSW
Lyle Cooper, PhD

INTRODUCTION

Appropriate treatments for many disorders, including adolescent substance abuse, have evolved over time. These changes may be driven by medical need or a breakthrough in technology, but are more often related to changes in the manner in which services are delivered, which in turn are driven by the importance that is placed on the disorder and the resources that are allocated to meeting the need. Adolescent substance abuse has not changed as dramatically as the services that have been developed to meet the needs over the last two decades.

Substance Use Among Adolescents

There are two primary national studies, which make annual estimates of adolescent substance use. The National Survey of Drug Use and Health is commissioned by the Substance Abuse and Mental Health Services Administration and utilizes a probability household sampling of all residents of the country regardless of age, and results for adolescents are drawn from the overall sample. The most recent available results (2005) suggest that 9.9 percent of youths aged 12 to 17 were current illicit drug users: 6.8 percent used marijuana, 3.3 percent used prescription-type drugs non-medically, 1.2 percent used inhalants, 0.8 percent used hallucinogens, and 0.6 percent used cocaine. Rates of current alcohol use were 4.2 percent among persons aged 12 or 13, 15.1 percent of persons aged 14 or 15, 30.1 percent of 16 or 17 year olds (NSDUH, 2007). The annual Monitoring the Future study funded by the National Institute of Drug Abuse and conducted by researchers at the University of Michigan also measures adolescent substance use. The study, which employs a school-based sampling of students in 8th, 10th and 12th grades, measures lifetime, annual, and current (30 day) use patterns reported not by age, but by grade level. Similar results were found by the study for current rates, however it is important to note that by 12th grade nearly three- fourths of students have used alcohol (72.7%) and almost half have used an illicit drug (48.2%) (Johnston, O'Malley, Bachman, and

Schulenberg, 2006). Thus suggesting that while many adolescents may use substances only a smaller portion will actually need treatment, and an even smaller portion will require residential services. For those individuals who are able to access substance abuse treatment services, the reported primary drugs of choice are marijuana (64%) followed by alcohol (19%) and stimulants (5%) (DASIS, 2006).

Need for Adolescent Substance Abuse Treatment

Currently, there is a significant need for substance abuse treatment for adolescents in the United States. Based on data from the National Surveys on Drug Use and Health (2007), the Office of Applied Studies at the Substance Abuse and Mental Health Services Administration (2006) was able to estimate the number of youth who needed substance abuse treatment, those who perceived a need for substance abuse treatment, those who received treatment, and the related treatment gap. Based on the National Survey on Drug Use and Health, one and a half million youths (6.1% youths aged 12 to 17) were classified as needing alcohol treatment in the past year and only about 111,000 youth (7.2% of those needing alcohol treatment) received specialty treatment for alcohol in the past year. Similarly, about one million, four hundred thousand youths (5.4%) were classified as needing illicit drug use treatment in the past year and 124,000 (9.1% of those needing illicit drug treatment) received specialty treatment for an illicit drug in the past year. Treatment access appears to be related to perceptions of a substance abuse problem. The same study found that youths who were in need of substance use treatment in the past year and did not receive treatment were not likely to perceive a need for substance use treatment. Only a small portion (15%) of adolescents who access substance abuse treatment services are currently able to access residential services (DASIS, 2006).

Efficacy of Adolescent Substance Abuse Treatment

Studies of adolescent substance abuse treatment generally do not show high levels of treatment retention, and individuals who complete services do not demonstrate high levels of abstinence following treatment, or high levels of pro-social behaviors post treatment (Rutherford and

Banta-Green, 1998; Muck, Zempolich, and Titus, 2001; Vaughn and Howard, 2004; Stevens and Moral, 2002). The majority of adolescents (58%-61%) who do access substance abuse treatment services do not complete services (OAS, 2007c). What is known substance abuse outcomes is that longer lengths of stay predict better outcomes (Hubbard, Craddock, Flynn, Anderson, and Etheridge, 1997), particularly for recipients of residential services (Greenfield, Burgdorf, Chen, Porowski, Roberts, and Harrell, 2004). Placement criteria developed by both the American Society of Addiction Medicine (2007), and the Center for Substance Abuse Treatment (1999) suggest that heavy using adolescents who are experiencing substance use problems should normally be referred to a residential level of care.

RECENT HISTORICAL TRENDS IN THE DELIVERY OF RESIDENTIAL SUBSTANCE ABUSE TREATMENT SERVICES TO ADOLESCENTS

Residential adolescent drug treatment has been found to be the most expensive modality of substance treatment services, costing $1,138 per week. In comparison adult residential costs were found to be $700 per week, and adolescent outpatient was $194 per week (Roebuck, French, and McLellan, 2003). Due to the high cost and previously mentioned relatively low outcomes for adolescent substance abuse treatment, residential services for substance using adolescents were one of the first targets of cost saving programs utilized by managed care organizations.

The late 1980s saw a dramatic shift in how services to adolescents were provided. As residential services were decreasing in the number of facilities, the number of beds in facilities, and the length of stay, service delivery methods began to evolve to meet the needs of the ever-changing environment. While the timeframe and intensity of services were set by the MCO's, the researchers/practitioners began to develop interventions to fit within the new framework, i.e., briefer interventions, a broader focus inclusive of mental health issues, a focus on evidence-based best practices.

There appears to be a new change on the horizon as residential substance abuse treatment services are being delivered increasingly outside of the domain of managed care organizations. It appears that individuals are more likely to self-pay, or more likely a parent or guardian will pay for residential services. One of the direct positive changes that occurred due to managed care is the increased awareness of mental health needs and ultimately the incorporation of mental health services with substance abuse services. It appears that residential services for adolescents are increasingly provided within mental health or integrated mental health/substance abuse facilities. Similarly as substance abuse services move away from health care and more towards criminal justice solutions, jails and prisons rather than hospitals and substance abuse treatment programs are increasingly delivering residential services.

Residential Substance Abuse Treatment in the Late 1980s

In 1988, Linda Sunshine and John Wright published a book on treatment centers entitled *The 100 best treatment centers for alcoholism and drug abuse* with the expressed aim of helping families who had been affected by alcoholism and/or drug abuse. The book was not intended to be a research instrument but does tout itself as being, "the only complete guide to the most outstanding rehabilitation facilities in the country" (Sunshine and Wright, 1988). As such, it offers a historical artifact providing a context against which the current substance abuse service delivery models can be contrasted. Service delivery to individuals with substance abuse problems has evolved substantially since the time when in patient or residential 45-day, Minnesota Model treatment centers were considered typical of best practice in the field for adolescents. The year 1988 represents a key date in substance abuse history, as after this date, the effects of managed care began to be felt by most facilities (Galanter, Keller, Dermatis, and Egelko, 1999). Thus, this paper explores the impact of health care system changes on substance abuse services during the transition to primarily a managed care system from primarily a fee for service insurance system, and through yet another transition to a reliance on self-pay.

Being that there were no established standardized objective criteria by which to judge the quality of the treatment centers, Sunshine and Wright (1988) developed criteria based on recommendations of professionals working in the field. These criteria provide an understanding of treatment standards in 1988 and the authors' intentions in determining what centers were included in the book. These standards included whether the facility:

- Offered at least 28 days' residential treatment;
- Was freestanding and devoted exclusively to addiction problems;
- Practiced the Minnesota Model, which was defined as a non-medical approach that includes: no drugs except during detoxification; the use of individual and group counseling geared to a self-help concept; the direct and continuous involvement of family members in treatment; the provision of aftercare; and treatment planning;
- Was committed to low staff turnover and a high degree of continuity of care;
- Promoted an Alcoholics Anonymous (AA) approach;
- Included family and after care services;
- Was staffed by well-trained administrators and program directors;
- Provided certified staff;
- Required 13 months' training for new employees and 3 months' training for experienced counselors; and
- Employed recovering counselors who were alcohol/drug free for four years (pp. 1-17).

Additionally, the authors recommended against individuals with substance use disorders seeking psychiatric treatment–at least initially–and suggested that, despite the relatively high costs of care (ranging then from $4,000 to more than $10,000 per episode), access to high quality care was possible, even for those in somewhat limited circumstances.

The Delivery of Substance Abuse Services Under Managed Care 1988-2003

For a fifteen year period, beginning in the late 1980s, health care, in general, and substance abuse treatment services, in particular, began to feel the effects of managed care. Managed care is often understood conceptually as a method of organizing health care service delivery and reimbursement. A common business strategy in managed care is to maximize outcomes at the lowest possible cost (Darby, 2007). The American

Medical Association (AMA) defines managed care as "those processes or techniques used by any entity that delivers, administers and/or assumes risk for health care services in order to control or influence the quality, accessibility, utilization or costs and prices or outcomes of such services provided to a defined enrollee population" (Bazelon Center, 2000). To better manage cost and quality, managed care organizations separated physical health from behavioral health through the use of specialized provider contracts known as carve outs.

Decreases in Private Dollars for Treatment

The impact of managed care and the decline in private insurance dollars for substance abuse treatment has greatly impacted substance abuse service delivery. Within a decade (1988-1998), three-quarters of monies spent by private insurance were cut. The value of addiction insurance coverage declined 74.5% between 1988 and 1998 for employees of mid-to large-size companies, as compared to a decline of 11.5% for general health care (Hay Group, 2000). This in turn created a shift from private dollars to public funding of substance abuse treatment. In 1987, private payers accounted for about 47% of all substance abuse treatment dollars, by 1997 public expenditures had increased to about 64% of all substance abuse treatment expenditures and private support had shrunk to about 36%. In particular, private insurance support for substance abuse treatment fell from about 32% in 1987 to approximately 24% in 1997 (SAMHSA, 2000). This decrease in funding led to a decrease in available services. In a study of residential substance abuse programs, researchers found a decline in number of days in treatment per episode down from 32.1 days in 1988 to 22.5 in 2001, while the average number of annual inpatient admissions rose from 834.7 in 1988 to over 1,033 in 2001 (MacMaster, Holleran, Chantus, and Kostyk, 2005).

Changes in Public Expenditures

With the emergence of public managed care for mental health and substance abuse treatment programs, states were challenged to stretch scarce public funds. Unlike the private sector, public mental health and substance abuse funding is disproportionate when compared to public expenditures for the same treatment. Public sector services receive government funding that tends to target sub-populations (mental illness or substance abuse), making it difficult for community programs to serve a broader and more diverse population. As a result local community service providers are forced to accept categorical funding targeted for specific individuals or for a specific type of treatment. As public payers struggle with diminishing budgets, quality of care is jeopardized for public consumers, who are relatively powerless to voice their concerns or influence policy or funding decisions (Darby, 2007).

Changes in "Best Practices"

Twenty-eight day, 12-step oriented programs are no longer considered to be best practice in the delivery of substance abuse services. Rather than using a single model for everyone, current best treatment practices focus on the delivery of highly individualized treatment that meets the multiple needs of individuals receiving substance abuse services. In comparison, a summary of a few of the most relevant principles for effective treatment, as outlined by the National Institute on Drug Abuse (2001) follows.

- Multiple treatment settings, interventions, and services that can be matched to each individual patient's particular problems and needs;
- Readily available treatment that attends to the multiple needs of the individual, including any associated medical, psychological, social, vocational, and legal problems;
- Continual assessment of an individual's treatment and services plan, modifying as necessary to ensure that the plan meets the person's changing needs, whether those needs be for medical services, family therapy, parenting instruction, vocational rehabilitation, or social and legal services;
- Strategies to engage and keep patients in treatment until the patient's threshold of significant recovery is reached, which, according to research, is reached at about 3 months (90 days) in treatment, after which point additional treatment will produce even further progress toward recovery; and

- Individual and or group counseling sessions as well as other behavioral therapies and, when necessary, medications used in conjunction with counseling.

DELIVERY OF RESIDENTIAL SUBSTANCE ABUSE SERVICES IN THE POST-MANAGED CARE ERA

It appears that there are three trends, which have occurred in the post-managed care era. At the anecdotal level, it appears that individuals are more likely to self-pay, or more likely a parent or guardian will pay for residential services. Secondly, it appears that one of the direct positive changes that occurred due to managed care is the increased awareness of mental health needs and ultimately the incorporation of mental health services with substance abuse services. It appears that residential services for adolescents are increasingly provided within mental health or integrated mental health/substance abuse facilities. The growth in integrated services has been tremendous. Thirdly, as substance abuse services move away from health care and more towards criminal justice solutions, jails and prisons rather than hospitals and substance abuse treatment programs are increasingly delivering residential services.

Self-Pay for Services

There is little evidence within the professional literature that individuals are increasingly self-paying for residential adolescent substance abuse services, however anecdotally the authors of this paper are of the opinion that this has increased dramatically. This change has set up a tiered system in which those individuals who can afford services are able to pay out of pocket for them, and those who do not have the means to do so do not have ready access to such services. Services at the high end of the spectrum remain often true to the Minnesota Model, although it is clear that these services have evolved over the last two decades. This leaves other potential service users of lesser means to rely on either their own managed health insurance resources, or on the public system which has increasing turned to integrated services and criminal justice solutions.

Residential Substance Abuse Services Within the Mental Health System

It is well known that many adolescents presenting to substance abuse treatment have co-occurring mental health needs (Grella, Hser, Joshi, and Rounds-Bryant, 2001). Increasingly however, rather stand alone residential substance abuse facilities individuals are increasingly finding access to this level of care within the mental health and not the substance abuse service system.

Substance Abuse Services Within the Criminal Justice System

The criminal justice system is the principal source of referral to treatment for the majority (52%) of youth who are admitted to substance abuse treatment (DASIS, 2006), which is in contrast to adults who are referred by the criminal justice system only about a third (36.3%) of the time (OAS, 2007b). However, the overall prevalence and availability of residential treatment for youth involved in the criminal justice system is relatively low (Young et al., 2007). For those individuals who were able to access and receive substance abuse treatment while incarcerated, treatment in a "residential setting" was primarily provided within the criminal justice institution that the individual was incarcerated. Data from the Uniform Facility Data Set (UFDS) and the Survey of Correctional Facilities found that about 80% of the 27,152 residents in juvenile facilities who received substance abuse treatment received their treatment in a general facility population setting. Less than a fifth, about 19%, received treatment in a specialized unit within a criminal justice facility, and about 1% received treatment in a specialized residential facility (OAS, 2007).

CONCLUSIONS

Residential substance abuse treatment for adolescents has experienced significant changes in recent years. Many of these changes have been driven by the advent of managed care. Three historical eras were conceptualized: (1) an era before the advent of managed care in which health insurance companies paid for longer stays on a fee for service basis,

(2) an era in which services were funded through managed care organizations and lengths of stay were significantly reduced, and (3) the current era in which residential services are primarily offered either through self-pay and other service systems. Practitioners who provide services to adolescents must be awareness of these changes and must respond with appropriate recommendations to their clients as well as advocacy on their behlf.

REFERENCES

American Society of Addiction Medicine. (2007). American Society of Addiction Medicine (ASAM) Second Edition–Revised of Patient Placement Criteria (ASAM PPC-2R).

Bureau of Justice Statistics (BJS). (2001). *Correctional population in the United States*. Washington DC: Bureau of Justice.

Center of Substance Abuse Treatment. (1999). Treatment of Adolescents with substance use disorders. Rockville, MD: Substance Abuse and Mental Health Services Administration.

Drug and Alcohol Services Information System (DASIS). (2006). Characteristics of Young Adult (Aged 18-25) and Youth (Aged 12-17) Admissions: 2004. Rockville, MD: Substance Abuse and Mental Health Services Administration.

Galanter, M., Keller, D. S., Dermatis, H., and Egelko, S. (1999). *The impact of managed care on addiction treatment: a problem in need of solution*. American Society of Addiction Medicine: Washington, DC.

Greenfield, L., Burgdorf, K., Chen, X., Porowski, A., Roberts, T., and Harrell, J. (2004). Effectiveness of long-term residential substance abuse treatment for women: findings from three national studies. American Journal of Drug and Alcohol Abuse, 30(3), 537-550.

Grella, C., Hser, Y., Joshi, V., and Rounds-Bryant, J. (2001). Drug treatment outcomes for adolescents with comorbid mental health and substance use disorders. Journal of Nervous and Mental Diseases, 189, 384-392.

Hubbard, R. L., Craddock, S. G., Flynn, P. M., Anderson, J., and Etheridge, R. M. (1997). Overview of 1-year follow-up outcomes in the Drug Abuse Treatment Outcome Study (DATOS). Psychology of Addictive Behaviors, 11(4), 261-278.

Johnston, L. D., O'Malley, P. M., Bachman, J. G., and Schulenberg, J. E. (2006). Teen drug use continues down in 2006, particularly among older teens; but use of prescription-type drugs remains high. University of Michigan News and Information Services: Ann Arbor, MI.

MacMaster, S. A., Holleran, L. K., Kostyk, L., and Chantus, D. (2005). Documenting Changes in the Delivery of Substance Abuse Services: The Status of the "100 Best Treatment Centers for Alcoholism and Drug Abuse" of 1988. Journal of Health and Social Policy, 20(3), 67-77.

Muck, R., Zempolich, K., and Titus, J. (2001). An overview of the effectiveness of adolescent substance abuse treatment models. Youth and Society, 33(2), 143-168.

National Institute on Drug Abuse (NIDA). (2001). *Principles of drug addiction treatment: A research-based guide*. NIDA: Washington, DC.

National Survey of Drug Use and Health (NSDUH). (2007). Results from the 2005 National Survey on Drug Use and Health: National Findings. Rockville, MD: Substance Abuse and Mental Health Services Administration.

Office of Applied Science. (2006). Substance Use Treatment Need among Adolescents 2003-2004. Rockville, MD: Substance Abuse and Mental Health Services Administration.

Office of Applied Science. (2007a). Substance Use Treatment in Adult and Juvenile Correctional Facilities. Rockville, MD: Substance Abuse and Mental Health Services Administration.

Office of Applied Science. (2007b). Treatment Episode Data Set (TEDS) Highlights-2005. Rockville, MD: Substance Abuse and Mental Health Services Administration.

Office of Applied Science. (2007c). Number of Discharges from Substance Abuse Treatment age 12 or older and Percent whq completed treatment course, United States, 2002-2004. Rockville, MD: Substance Abuse and Mental Health Services Administration.

Roebuck, M., French, M., and McLellan, T. (2003). DATStats: Results from 85 studies using the Drug Abuse Treatment Cost Analysis Program (DATCAP). Journal of Substance Abuse Treatment, 25, 51-57.

Rutherford, M., and Banta-Green, C. (1998). Effectiveness standards for the treatment of chemical dependency in juvenile offenders: A review of the literature. Seattle: University of Washington, Alcohol and Drug Institute.

Rydell, C. P., and Everingham, S. S. (1994). Controlling cocaine: supply versus demand programs. Prepared for the Office of National Drug Control Policy and the United States Army. Drug Policy Research Center, Rand Corporation: Santa Monica, CA.

Stevens, S., and Moral, A. (2002). Adolescent substance abuse treatment in the United States: Exemplary models from a national evaluation study. Binghamton, NY: Haworth Press.

Substance Abuse and Mental Health Services Administration (SAMHSA). (1999). *Summary of outcomes in the national treatment improvement evaluation study, NEDS fact sheet 4, 1997*. Rockville, MD: SAMHSA.

Substance Abuse and Mental Health Services Administration (SAMHSA). (1999). *Uniform Facility Data Set Survey (UFDS), 1995-1997*. SAMHSA: Rockville, MD.

Sunshine, L., and Wright, J. W. (1988). *The 100 best treatment centers for alcoholism and drug abuse*. Avon: New York, New York.

Vaughn M., and Howard, M. (2004). Adolescent substance abuse treatment: A synthesis of controlled evaluations. Research on Social Work Practice, 14, 325-335.

Young, D., Dembo, R., and Henderson, C. (2007). A national survey of substance abuse treatment for juvenile offenders. Journal of Substance Abuse Treatment, 32, 255-266.

Effecting Successful Community Re-Entry: Systems of Care Community Based Mental Health Services

Rebecca I. Estes, PhD, OTR/L, ATP
Claudette Fette, OTR, CRC
Marjorie E. Scaffa, PhD, OTR/L, FAOTA

INTRODUCTION

The need for system reform for child and adolescent mental health services was documented as early as 1930, re-emerged throughout the 1960s, 1970s and continues into the current decade (Meyers, 1985; Collins & Collins, 1994; Stroul, 2003; Knitzer, 2005). Children with mental health needs often do not receive services or receive excessively restrictive or inappropriate services; the services may be limited to facility based treatments or occur in fragmented systems, restricting successful community re-entry, and they often lack in cultural competence and concern (Stroul, 2003; Knitzer, 2005). The 1978 President's Commission on Mental Health identified children and adolescents with serious emotional disturbances as an underserved population; the Commission's report led to the passage of the 1981 Mental Health System Act which authorized funds for identification, needs assessment, and provision and coordination of services to children with mental illness (Meyers, 1985). After a year of planning and development of programs to create local systems, the law was repealed and replaced by the Alcohol, Drug Abuse and Mental Health Block Grant Program which shifted control of federal money to the state and did not target funds for mental health services for children (Meyers, 1985).

Jane Knitzer released her Children's Defense Fund supported report, *Unclaimed Children*, in 1982, documenting the poor state of services for severely emotionally disturbed children and adolescents and fostering a movement that created "system of care." interagency mental health delivery systems with a family focus (Knitzer, 2005). The Child and Adolescent Service System Program (CASSP) evolved out of the systems of care movement and was created in 1984 to assure that children with the most severe mental health needs would get what they required without having to go through child welfare, juvenile justice or special education services. CASSP centered on the concept of systems of care which calls for multi-agency coordination of services that are community based, child centered, and family centered. The goals of CASSP were to ensure that the mental health needs of children and their families were met through interagency systems, to increase mental health agency involvement in the systems of care agencies, to increase the families' role, and to increase the cultural competence of services provided (Lourie & Hernandez, 2003). It supported the creation of the parent movement and the shift toward family members serving major roles in development and running of systems of care based programs rather than pitting systems against families as contributors to the problem.

In 2003, the President's New Freedom Commission released its report "Achieving the Promise: Transforming Mental Health Care in America." The commission was given the charge of identifying the problems in the mental health delivery systems and making concrete recommendations for improvement to ". . . allow adults with serious mental illness and children with serious emotional disturbance to live, work, learn, and participate fully in their communities" (Hogan, 2003, p. 1467). The report lays out six goals, each with specific recommendations to reorient mental health systems toward recovery. The New Freedom Commission goals are that in a transformed mental health system:

1. Americans understand that mental health is essential to overall health,
2. mental health care is consumer and family driven,
3. disparities in mental health services are eliminated,
4. early mental health screening, assessment, and referral to services are common practice,
5. excellent mental health care is delivered and research is accelerated, and
6. technology is used to access mental health care and information" (Hogan, 2003, p. 1470).

In the 2003 Commission report, opportunities for systems of care based community reentry programs emerge as consumer and family driven treatment and school based mental health models are supported as is the need for research, evidence based practices and an improved workforce. The commission report has been used to retool funding priorities for the United States Substance Abuse and Mental Health Services Administration and serves as the basis for the federal Mental Health Transformation grants.

SYSTEMS OF CARE

The core values of the systems of care philosophy are that systems must be child centered and family focused, community based, and culturally competent (http://systemsofcare.samhsa.gov). Principles applicable to community reentry as well as community based programs with a focus on early identification and prevention include comprehensiveness, individualization, least restrictive setting, family orientation, service integration, case management, early identification, smooth transition, rights protection and advocacy and nondiscrimination. Development of systems of care programs occurs at the local level with changes in policies and funding that allow for planning, implementing and evaluating service delivery of coordinated mental health services and supports across systems to support individually designed service plans that support children and families in their community (Day & Roberts, 1991). As these are individually determined systems, the inherent challenge is to understand the relationships between variables at the system level and at the practice level.

Family-driven principles are featured in both systems of care and the New Freedom Commission documents. Family involvement, a vital element in transforming mental health systems, requires a deliberate effort on the part of systems and service providers and must be the organizing concept in systems of care reforms (Huffine & Anderson, 2003). Family advocates, or partners, are composed of families who raised children with behavioral disorders and then assumed volunteer or professional roles in supporting other families with children with behavioral disorders, providing practical advice, support from common experience and systems advocacy. Key features of this role include listening, affirming strengths and competencies, maintaining a supportive relationship and facilitating opportunities for families with children with mental, emotional or behavioral disorders to provide mutual assistance and ongoing coaching (Huffine & Anderson, 2003; Ireys, Devet & Sakwa, 2002). In a systems of care program that is functioning well, family advocates are involved at all levels, from family-to-family advocacy to program planning, training and governance.

Increasing family partnership and empowerment in family groups increases outcomes, satisfaction and self advocacy through building parent to parent support (Carrigan, Rodger & Copley, 2001; Christie & Hedayati, 2003). Supportive environments mediate the impact of stress on psychological wellbeing by providing a sense of belonging, support and coping resources, acceptance and opportunities for empowerment and advocacy (Law, King, Stewart, & King, 2001). Rebeiro (2001) stressed the importance of creating affirming environments that create opportunity to be with one's "own," to enable a sense of equity and commonality, self expression in safety, and a focus on strengths and abilities. These are an important counter to the stigma and identification of negatives that dominates the experience of many families living with mental illness and establishes a foundation for the provision of value-based practice, interventions that are consistent with recovery values (Farkas & Anthony, 2006).

Interventions and approaches must also be evidence based and while some research results are available, additional research is needed on promoting recovery and resiliency as well as mechanisms for prevention and cures for mental illness (Hogan, 2003). Key outcomes reported for the Comprehensive Community Mental Health Services Program for Children and Their Families encompassed cost savings, client based improvements and better placement outcomes (Substance Abuse and Mental Health Service Administration [SAMHSA], 2006). The program resulted in $2,776.85 average per child cost savings over 12 months due to reduced inpatient hospital days; additionally, there was a 54% decrease in the number of children who used inpatient facilities resulting in an average cost savings of $784.16 per child. Implementation of the program resulted in client based improvements including a reduction in the number of arrests per child, increased emotional and behavioral stability for almost 90% of the children in systems of care after 18 months, and a 32% reduction in the number of children who had suicide related behaviors after 12 months in the program. The percent of children regularly attending school improved to 84% and overall academic performance improved to 75% children passing after 18 months in systems of care. Improved placement outcomes were seen in the 43% decrease in juvenile detention or other secure facilities (SAMHSA, 2006). These data provide initial evidence to support the viability of the systems of care approach for community reentry; however, further studies need to be conducted to provide both evidence-based and value-based data.

COLLABORATION OF DISCIPLINES– "IT TAKES A VILLAGE . . ."

Chenven and Brady defined collaboration, tongue in cheek, as ". . . an unpleasurable activity performed by nonconsenting adults in public" (2003, p. 79). A more workable definition is that ". . . collaboration is ultimately about people solving real problems and achieving meaningful outcomes through cooperative work. At its core, collaboration facilitates the solving of a problem situation in a new way that actively recognizes and accommodates to both the strengths and the needs of all involved in the work process" (Chenven & Brady, 2003, p. 80). Collaboration is required in a systems of care approach to ensure success. Creation of a caring "village" entails collaboration and cooperation among disciplines as well as agencies and must be embraced as a systemic value and process (vertically and horizontally within and across organizations) and true partnership with youth and families. The creation of a successful "village" depends on reliable and trusting relationships and is most difficult in the earliest stages when disciplines and partners don't understand each other's training, responsibilities, mandates and resource bases. When a systems of care program at this stage of development is faced with challenges, staff may split, blame and become defensive. Development must occur at the clinical, management and support staff levels to assure commitment to the creation of multidisciplinary, multi-agency teamwork and system building.

Community based systems of care programs often must invest additional resources in training entry level staff because health professionals continue to be prepared in traditional university systems that focus more on medical models. Basic competencies for all disciplines working with community based and community reentry systems of care programs include capability for collaborative work with families and a fundamental understanding that rather than being the problem, families are part of the solution. Greater awareness is needed of what contributions the diverse health related disciplines can contribute to a successful "village." The breadth of child serving agencies and their roles within the network must be broadly known in order for cross disciplinary collaboration and networking to occur. Successful reentry and on-going community involvement of families and children with mental health needs requires understanding of and skill in identification and use of nonprofessional, natural community supports; sensitivity and basic understanding of cultural differences and culturally competent practices; and knowledge of wraparound facilitation and evidence based practices in children's mental health.

Essential training for any professionals working in a systems of care program has been identified and categorized into three areas through work done at the Pennsylvania CASSP Training and Technical Assistance Institute (McGinty, Diamond, Brown, & McCammon, 2003). The first area identified is child, family and community core competencies which includes basic knowledge of development, diagnostic criteria and effective practices. Second, is training in strategies to work effectively with families as partners. The third area is training in research and program evaluation and should include exposure to a variety of research methodologies to evaluate practice. The authors also offer suggestions for implementing training initiatives to retool the provider base adequately. They suggest integration of systems of care philosophy into existing curricula with inclusion of parents of children with serious emotional disturbance as faculty and use of interdisciplinary faculty collaboration. Systems of care experience needs to become part of fieldwork training with specific attention given to processing the differences between traditional services and systems of care philosophy in the following six areas: (1) partnering with families, (2) attending to caregiver stress, (3) service planning, (4) interdisciplinary collaboration, (5) outcomes and accountability, and (6) supervision (McGinty et al., 2003). Opportunities for systems of care rotations in fieldwork are limited but seeking out partnerships with existing systems of care programs as well as with family organizations that practice the principles of systems of care provide rich opportunities for experiencing the distinct differences in systems.

Disciplines traditionally trained in programs with a medical model focus have a long way to go to prepare and to embrace the flexible, multidisciplinary team with its blended roles described above. Occupational therapy has traditionally practiced in a medical or rehabilitation context; however, emerging practice areas includes community based practice. A challenge for occupational therapy, as with other disciplines, is crossing the barriers to a collaborative interdisciplinary systems of care approach. A first step is knowledge and sharing information about the potential contributions and skills each team member can bring to the "village." The following sections are provided in an attempt to initiate the sharing of information across disciplines by by discussing the potential contributions and skills that occupational therapists bring to a systems of care village.

THE ROLE OF OCCUPATIONAL THERAPY IN COMMUNITY AND SYSTEMS OF CARE

Although occupational therapy and systems of care share similar philosophical principles and have common goals, there are few references to occupational therapy in the systems of care literature. Occupational therapists have a unique skill set to facilitate the successful participation of children and youth with psychosocial needs in the community. Occupational therapists currently provide services to children in a variety of settings including hospitals, foster care, home health, residential facilities and schools. Roles for occupational therapists that are particularly applicable to community practice within the systems of care context include case manager, multidisciplinary team member and consultant. The role of occupational therapy in child and adolescent mental health, family-centered care, residential care and community integration, and school-based intervention will be described here to illustrate the many contributions occupational therapy can make to systems of care based programs for children and adolescents with mental health needs.

Child and Adolescent Mental Health

The roots of occupational therapy are firmly grounded in psychiatry and the moral treatment movement. In 1917, the initial founders of the profession included a psychiatrist, a social worker, a teacher and a nurse (Bing, 1981). Occupational therapy's unique area of expertise is its knowledge of occupation (daily life activities) and how engagement in occupation can be used to improve human performance and ameliorate the disabling effects of illness or injury. Occupational therapists address the psychosocial factors that impact occupational performance and function in activities of daily living, work, school, play, leisure and social participation. The psychosocial factors of interest include, but are not limited to, cognition, emotional expression, interpersonal skills, social behaviors and social support. In addition, an "interruption in a person's ability to engage in and succeed at necessary and valued daily occupations elicits emotional and psychological responses that are central to how the person responds and eventually adapts" (American Occupational Therapy Association [AOTA], 2005, p. 5). The goal of therapy is to restore, maintain and improve function for persons with physical and mental limitations, and to prevent injury and promote health. Using everyday life activities and occupations, occupational therapy enables persons with mental illness to enhance their role competence, satisfaction and quality of life in personal care, employment, education, and community living (Jackson & Arbesman, 2005; AOTA, 2006).

In mental health, occupational therapy utilizes a biopsychosocial framework and a strengths-based approach to promote recovery and build resilience. The occupational therapist engages the child's interest in activities and occupations in order to facilitate improved function, rather than focusing on the diagnosis or disorder solely (Gray, 2005). As experts in child development, occupational therapists are able to incorporate appropriate developmental tasks in the therapy process. A literature review of occupation-based articles in children's mental health found that successful practices shared some common features including:

1. direct instruction toward targeted skills;
2. activities to teach and encourage practice of new skills;
3. peers to model and promote practice of new skills;

4. a supportive adult to provide coaching and reinforcement for appropriate behavior; and
5. a sufficient length of time to provide ample intervention and practice-emergent skills (Jackson & Arbesman, 2005, p. 31-32).

Occupational therapists working with children with behavioral disorders have developed intervention strategies addressing coping and sensory processing capacity as well as strategies to foster occupational development and performance particularly within peer and family groups (Olson, 2001). The overall goal of these interventions is to help clients "use time and their environments to use or create opportunities for activity in a personally meaningful way that leads to their successful participation in their occupational roles . . . (which for children are) being a student, a friend, a player, a son or daughter, a worker" (Olson, 2001, p 174). Studies within occupational therapy literature demonstrate the effectiveness of active participation in social and achievement occupations in adolescence to increase coping, general and school satisfaction and intrinsic motivation. More research is needed within the profession to support children's occupations in naturally occurring environments and to study playfulness and predictive leisure experiences (Farnworth, 2000; Hess & Bundy, 2003; Passmore, 2003).

Family Centered Care

Currently, occupational therapists are not integral members of the systems of care team. Yet, the fit is evident in recent occupational therapy literature that speaks to the idea of collaboration with families within the context of family involvement in individual treatment processes and planning activities (Andersson, 2004; Wooster, 2001; Hanna & Rodger, 2002). Family centered care in occupational therapy is grounded in the assumption that parents know what is best for their child; it conceptualizes families as partners with providers; families collaborate to determine what is essential to work on and therapists provide information and instruction that parents designate as important to them (Wooster, 2001; Andersson, 2004). Assumptions underlying successful collaboration are that

1. the unit of intervention is the family,
2. diversity is celebrated,

3. services are flexible and responsive to the family,
4. decision making is best done in partnership, and
5. wider community resources should be incorporated (Hanna & Rodger, 2002).

In addition, occupational therapists may facilitate family mental health. For example, they can support creation of special family rituals and routines around meaningful activities (Werner DeGrace, 2003) and opportunities to participate in real life situations that enable children to build the knowledge, skills and capacity to interact, work and live with others (Bednell, Cohn & Dumas, 2005). Children with disabilities generally and particularly those with behavioral disorders and their families are restricted in active recreation, community participation, socialization, and normative childhood occupations (Bednell et al., 2005; Cronin, 2004). Research on the experience of raising children with mental, emotional and behavioral disorders reveals that families feel isolated, frustrated, exhausted and overwhelmed, and undergo stigma, grieving and increased fragmentation in the quality of their occupations (Cronin, 2004; Donovan, VanLeit, Crowe & Keefe, 2005; Helitzer, Cunningham-Sabo, VanLeit & Crowe, 2002). Adaptive family routines can protect health by providing stabilization, family identity and support for wellbeing of members under stress (Werner Degrace, 2003).

Residential Care and Community Integration

Although the general public tends to identify occupational therapy with medical facilities, particularly rehabilitation hospitals, the profession has a long history in residential care and home health. Occupational therapists work in group homes, halfway houses, apartment complexes for persons with special needs, assisted living facilities, and other types of supportive housing. Occupational therapy in supportive housing for persons with mental illness can take many forms. A home management program in New Jersey focused on teaching consumers the skills necessary to manage their homes safely and effectively. The program components consisted of care and cleaning of the home, safety issues, simple home repairs, decorating and use of community resources (Nolan & Swarbrick, 2002). Although other professionals can conduct home management training, occupational therapists are particularly qualified to provide this service, as home management is an instrumental activity of daily living within the profession's scope of practice. In addition, occupational therapists are trained in task analysis, and adaptation and modification of tasks and environments to enhance function.

As a complement to direct services to consumers, occupational therapists can provide program consultation and training for housing program staff members. This involves assisting direct care workers improve the ways they support consumers' development of ADL and socialization skills. In-service training topics typically include grooming and hygiene, socialization, community mobility, sexual health, home management, money management, safety and medication routine (Zimmerman, 1999).

Safe, secure housing contributes to the quality of life and health of persons with mental illness, but housing by itself is not adequate. Children and adults with mental illness need flexible and adjustable support services to enable them to improve and maintain functional status, prevent relapse and successfully adapt to community living. Supports must be tailored to the individual's needs and accommodate to fluctuating changes in function over time. Occupational therapists by virtue of their training can be instrumental in determining what supports are needed to optimally sustain persons in the community (Fossey, Harvey, Plant & Pantelis, 2006).

Community reentry and community integration involve an analysis of the person's capability to perform necessary tasks, analysis of the skills needed for those tasks, adaptation of the environment and identification of supports to enable functioning, and development of skill building strategies (Scheinholtz, 2001). Occupational therapists are particularly skilled at matching contextual characteristics with the needs and abilities of the person in order to determine the most appropriate and least restrictive environments in which individuals can participate successfully.

School-Based Intervention

For children and adolescents, school participation and performance are critical facilitators of development. School systems now employ large numbers of occupational therapists, and although they typically serve children with physical and learning disabilities, school-based occupational therapists are well trained to address the needs of children and adolescents with mental, emotional and behavioral disorders and their families.

School readiness is not simply a function of cognitive ability; numerous studies have indicated that behavioral and psychosocial skills are a good predictor of academic success. These skills include following teacher instructions, getting along with others, making friends, identifying and appropriately expressing emotions, delaying gratification, sharing, responding to feedback, and controlling impulses (Jackson & Arbesman, 2005). All of these skills are learned and modified through participation in occupations, and therefore can be remediated through occupational therapy.

Unfortunately, many students with emotional disturbances who could benefit from occupational therapy do not receive services. This is frequently due to a lack of understanding on the part of parents and educators regarding the professional role, expertise and scope of practice of occupational therapists. If psychosocial needs are identified and incorporated into the student's Individualized Education Plan (IEP), then occupational therapy can be provided (Jackson & Arbesman, 2005). Emotional disturbances are defined by the Individuals with Disabilities Education Act as:

> . . . a condition exhibiting one or more of the following characteristics over a long period of time and to a marked degree that adversely affects a child's educational performance—
>
> A. An inability to learn that cannot be explained by intellectual, sensory, or health factors.
> B. An inability to build or maintain satisfactory interpersonal, relationships with peers and teachers.
> C. Inappropriate types of behavior or feelings under normalc ircumstances.
> D. A general pervasive mood of unhappiness or depression.
> E. A tendency to develop physical symptoms or fears associated with personal or school problems." (National Dissemination Center for Children with Disabilities, 2004, p. 1)

Children with emotional disturbances often have difficulty with following directions, regulating their behavior, interpersonal relationships, participating in group activities and communication (Barnes, Beck, Vogel, Grice & Murphy, 2003).

Research indicates that the performance areas most often addressed by occupational therapists working with children with emotional disturbances in the schools include: handwriting, computer skills, play/recreation, communication and student role performance. In addition, specific skill areas addressed are fine motor dexterity, attention span, self-control, organizational skills and managing transitions. Children are treated individually and in groups using a variety of modalities including sensory integration, sensorimotor activities, schoolwork tasks, facilitation of adaptation, environmental modification, play and social activities (Barnes, Beck, Vogel, Grice & Murphy, 2003).

An emerging area for occupational therapy practice in the school system is in transition planning. Transition planning and intervention services prepare students with disabilities who are leaving secondary school for independent living, employment and community participation. Transition services are included in IDEA 97 and typically consist of community living objectives, instruction, support services, vocational evaluation, development of independent living skills, and community experiences (Kardos & White, 2006). Occupational therapists have found the occupation-based Assessment of Motor and Process Skills (AMPS) and the Allen Cognitive Levels screen (ACL-90) to be particularly useful in predicting post-secondary school transition needs and successful community integration (Kardos & White, 2006; Lee, Gargiullo, Brayman, Kinsey, Jones & Shotwell, 2003).

CONCLUSION

The New Freedom Commission's focus on recovery of ability to live, work, play, learn and participate in community reinforces the role of occupational therapists in providing valuable community supports for children and adolescents with mental health needs (Gray, 2005). Occupational therapy is an essential component of the mental health evaluation and intervention process for persons of all ages with mental disorders (American Occupational Therapy Association, 2006) and therefore has a role in systems of care based programs for children and adolescents with psychosocial needs. Occupational therapists can become part of the systems of care based programs through their roles in schools, residential settings, health care agencies, and community organizations.

Occupational therapists facilitate competence by using their expertise in task analysis, activity design, child development and adaptive functioning to facilitate engagement in just right challenges in support of increased adaptive behaviors. The identification of areas of success and problems, barriers and supports for occupational performance, contexts, occupational history and child and family's desired outcomes as part of an occupational profile is the initial step in evaluation (Jackson & Arbesman, 2005). Occupational therapy intervention can facilitate adaptive responses by individuals, families, systems and communities. These distinctive abilities further validate occupational therapists as valuable members of the systems of care team.

There is a need for increased communication among disciplines in order to fully understand and utilize the skills and strengths of team members who have the potential for valuable contributions toward a systems of care village. Interdisciplinary team members must thoughtfully design and implement research collaboratively with one another and family organizations that identifies child and family needs for successful reentry and participation in community and then, again collaboratively, to develop, implement and document the efficacy of community based interventions to meet the identified needs. The commonalities of philosophy and goals of occupational therapy and systems of care make the partnership particularly exciting.

REFERENCES

American Occupational Therapy Association (AOTA). (2006). *AOTA's statement on mental health practice.* Bethesda: Author.

Andersson, E. (2004). *Occupational adaptation: Assessing families' adaptive capacity.* Unpublished doctoral dissertation, Texas Woman's University, Denton, Texas.

Barnes, K.J., Beck, A.J., Vogel, K.A., Grice, K.O., & Murphy, D. (2003). Perceptions regarding school-based occupational therapy for children with emotional disturbances. *American Journal of Occupational Therapy, 57*(3), 337-341.

Bednell, G.M., Cohn, E.S., & Dumas, H.M. (2005). Exploring parents' use of strategies to promote social participation of school-age children with acquired brain injuries. *American Journal of Occupational Therapy, 59,* 273-284.

Bing, R.K. (1981). Occupational therapy revisited: A paraphrastic journey. *American Journal of Occupational Therapy, 35,* 499-518.

Carrigan, N., Roger, S., & Copley, J. (2001). Parent satisfaction with a paediatric occupational therapy service: pilot investigation. *Physical and Occupational Therapist in Pediatrics, 21, 51-76.*

Chenven, M., & Brady, B. (2003). Collaboration across disciplines and among agencies within systems of care. In Pumariega, A.J. & Winters, N.C. (Eds.), *The Handbook of Child and Adolescent Systems of Care, The New Community Psychiatry* (pp. 66-81). San Francisco: Jossey-Bass.

Christie, A., & Hedayati, L. (2003). A programme for parents of children with challenging behaviors: An occupational therapy approach. *New Zealand Journal of Occupational Therapy, 50,* 11-16.

Collins, B.G., & Collins, M.C. (Jan/Feb 1994). Child and adolescent mental health: Building a system of care. *Journal of Counseling & Development, 72,* 239-243.

Cronin, A.F. (2004). Mothering a child with hidden impairments. *American Journal of Occupational Therapy, 58,* 83-92.

Day, C., & Roberts, M.C. (1991). Activities of the child and adolescent service system program for improving mental health services for children and families. *Journal of Clinical Child Psychology, 20*(4), 340-350.

Donovan, J.M., VanLeit, B.J., Crowe, T.K., & Keefe, E.B. (2005). Occupational goals of mothers of children with disabilities: influence of temporal, social and emotional contexts. *American Journal of Occupational Therapy, 59,* 249-261.

Farkas, M., & Anthony, W.A. (2006). System transformation through best practices. *Psychiatric Rehabilitation Journal, 30*(2), 87-88. Retrieved February 17, 2007, from the EBSCOhost Research Databases.

Farnworth, L. (2000). Time use and leisure occupations of young offenders. *American Journal of Occupational Therapy, 54,* 315-325.

Fossey, E., Harvey, C., Plant, G., & Pantelis, C. (2006). Occupational performance of people diagnosed with schizophrenia in supported housing and outreach programmes in Australia. *British Journal of Occupational Therapy, 69*(9), 409-419.

Gray, K. (2005). Mental illness in children and adolescents: A place for occupational therapy. *Mental Health Special Interest Section Quarterly, 28*(2), 1-3.

Hanna, K., & Rodger, S. (2002). Towards family-centered practice in paediatric occupational therapy: A review of the literature on parent-therapist collaboration. *Australian Journal of Occupational Therapy, 49,* 14-24.

Helitzer, D.L., Cunningham-Sabo, L.D., VanLeit B., & Crowe, T.K. (2002). Perceived changes in self-image and coping strategies of mothers of children with disabilities. *Occupational Therapy Journal of Research, 22,* 25-33.

Hess, L.M., & Bundy, A.C. (2003). The association between playfulness and coping in adolescents. *Physical and Occupational Therapy in Pediatrics, 23*(2), 5-17.

Hogan, M.F. (2003). The president's new freedom commission: Recommendations to transform mental health in America. *Psychiatric Services, 54*(11), 1467-1474. Downloaded February 17, 2007 from: http://ps.psychiatryonline.org

Huffine, C., & Anderson, D. (2003). Family advocacy development in systems of care. In Pumariega, A.J. & Winters, N.C. (Eds.), *The Handbook of Child and Adolescent*

Systems of Care, The New Community Psychiatry (pp. 35-65). San Francisco: Jossey-Bass.

Ireys, H.T., Devet, K.A., & Sakwa, D. (2002). Family support and education. In Burns, J. & Hoagwood, K. (Eds.), *Community Treatment for Youth* (pp. 154-176). NY: Oxford University Press.

Jackson, L.L., & Arbesman, M. (2005). *Occupational therapy practice guidelines for children with behavioral and psychosocial needs*. Bethesda: American Occupational Therapy Association.

Kardos, M.R., & White, B.P. (2006). Evaluation options for secondary transition planning. *American Journal of Occupational Therapy, 60*(3), 333-339.

Knitzer, J. (2005). Advocacy for children's mental health: *A personal journey. Journal of Clinical Child and Adolescent Psychology, 34*(4), 612-618.

Law, M., King, S., Stewart, D., & King, G. (2001). The perceived effects of parent-led support groups for parents of children with disabilities. *Physical and Occupational Therapy in Pediatrics, 21*, 29-48.

Lee, S.N., Gargiullo, A., Brayman, S., Kinsey, J.C., Jones, H.C., & Shotwell, M. (2003). Adolescent performance on the Allen cognitive Levels Screen. *American Journal of Occupational Therapy, 57*(3), 342-356.

Lourie, I.S., & Hernandez, M. (2003). A historical perspective on national child mental health policy. *Journal of Emotional and Behavioral Disorders, 11*(1), 5-9.

McGinty, K.L., Diamond, J.M., Brown, M.B., & McCammon, S.L. (2003). Training child and adolescent psychiatrists and child mental health professionals for systems of care. In Pumariega, A.J. & Winters, N.C. (Eds.), *The Handbook of Child and Adolescent Systems of Care, The New Community Psychiatry* (pp. 487-507). San Francisco: Jossey-Bass.

Meyers, J.C. (1985). Federal efforts to improve mental health services for children: Breaking a cycle of failure. *Journal of Clinical Child Psychiatry, 14*(3), 182-187.

National Dissemination Center for Children with Disabilities. (2004). Emotional disturbance fact sheet 5. Retrieved March 19, 2007 from http://www.nichcy.org/pubs/factshe/fs5txt.htm

Nolan, C., & Swarbrick, P. (2002). Supportive housing occupational therapy home management program. *Mental Health Special Interest Section Quarterly, 25*(2), 1-3.

Olson, L.J. (2001). Child psychiatry in the USA. In Lougher, L. (Ed.), *Occupational Therapy for Child and Adolescent Mental Health* (pp. 173-191). London: Churchill Livingstone.

Passmore, A. (2003). The occupation of leisure: Three typologies and their influence on mental health in adolescents. *Occupational Therapy Journal of Research, 23*, 76-84.

Rebeiro, K.L. (2001). Enabling occupation: The importance of an affirming environment. *Canadian Journal of Occupational Therapy, 68*, 80-89.

Stroul, B. (2003). Systems of care. In Pumariega, A.J. & Winters, N.C. (Eds.), *The Handbook of Child and Adolescent Systems of Care, The New Community Psychiatry* (pp. 17-34). San Francisco: Jossey-Bass.

Substance Abuse and Mental Health Service Administration. (May 2006). *SAMHSA News Release: Community-Based Care Leads to Meaningful Improvement for Children and*

Youth with Serious Mental Health Needs. Downloaded February 14, 2007 from: http://systemsofcare.samhsa.gov/news/nrindex.aspx

Werner Degrace, B. (2003). The issue is–Occupation-based and family-centered care: A challenge for current practice. *American Journal of Occupational Therapy, 54,* 347-350.

Wooster, D.A. (2001). Early intervention programs. In Scaffa, M. (Ed.), *Occupational Therapy in Community-Based Practice Settings* (pp. 280-283). Philadelphia: F.A. Davis Company.

Zimmerman, S.S. (1999). Occupational therapy service delivery to an apartment program. *Home and Community Health Special Interest Section Quarterly, 6*(1), 1-4.

About the Contributors

Michael L. Burford, MSSW, is a PhD Student at the College of Social Work, The University of Tennessee.

Lyle Cooper, PhD, LCSW, earned his degree in Social Work from Spalding University. He is Assistant Professor at the College of Social Work, The University of Tennessee. He is also a Licensed Clinical Social Worker and a Certified Alcohol and Drug Counselor.

Gary D. Ellis, PhD, earned his degree in higher education administration from the University of North Texas. He is currently Professor in the Department of Parks, Recreation and Tourism at the University of Utah.

Rebecca I. Estes, PhD, OTR/L, ATP, earned her degree in Occupational Therapy from Texas Women's University. She is Associate Professor and Chair, Department of Occupational Therapy, University of South Alabama.

Claudette Fette, OTR, CRC, is Founder of the Denton County Federation of Families in Denton County, TX.

Tammy Holmes, MA, earned her degree in Educational Psychology and Counseling Education from Tennessee Technological University. She is the Drug Court Coordinator for the Upper Cumberland Juvenile Drug Court, employed through the Upper Cumberland Community Service Agency.

Carole Lovell, PsyD, MSSW, LCSW, earned her PsyD from Southern California University for Professional Studies and her MSSW from the University of Tennessee. Licensed as a Clinical Social Worker in Tennesse, she is also the Program Director for the Personal Growth and Learning Center in Cookeville, TN.

Samuel A. MacMaster, PhD, MSSA, earned his degrees from Case Western Reserve University. He is Associate Professor at the College of Social Work, The University of Tennessee.

William R. Nugent, PhD, MSSW, earned his degrees from Florida State University. He is Professor and Director of the Doctoral Program at the College of Social Work, The University of Tennessee, Knoxville.

Marjorie E. Scaffa, PhD, OTR/L, FAOTA, earned her degree in Health Education from the University of Maryland. She is Professor at the Department of Occupational Therapy, the University of South Alabama.

Karen M. Sowers, PhD, is Dean and Professor at the University of Tennessee College of Social Work in Knoxville.

Lori K. Holleran Stiker, PhD, MSW, ACSW, earned her PhD from Arizona State University and a MSW from the University of Pennsylvania. She is Associate Professor in the School of Social Work at the University of Texas, Austin.

Gregory Washington, PhD, MSW, LCSW, earned his degrees from Clark Atlanta University. He is Associate Professor at the University of Tennessee at Martin.

Jerry Watson, PhD, earned his degree in Urban Higher Education from Jackson State University. He is Assistant Vice President and Director of Housing and e-City Development for Jackson State University.

Roderick J. Watts, PhD, earned his degree from the University of Maryland, College Park. He is Associate Professor of Psychology at Georgia State University. He is also a member of the Community and Clinical Psychology Program

John Wodarski, PhD, MSSW, earned his PhD from Washington University and a MSSW from The University of Tennessee. He is Professor at the College of Social Work at The University of Tennessee.

Julie Worley, FNP, PMHNP, holds a Masters Degree in family practice from University of Illinois Chicago and a psychiatric nurse practitioner degree from University of South Alabama. She is a Family and Psychiatric Mental Health Nurse Practitioner with fifteen years experience as an advanced practice nurse and ten prior years experience as an RN. She is affiliated with the Personal Growth and Learning Center in Cookesville, TN.

Erik Yost, MS, earned his degree from the University of Utah. He also holds a BFA in advertising design from Syracuse University.

Index

Numbers followed by t indicate tables.